The Five Series Study

MORTALITY OF MILITARY PARTICIPANTS IN U.S. NUCLEAR WEAPONS TESTS

Medical Follow-up Agency
INSTITUTE OF MEDICINE
by
Susan Thaul,
William F. Page,
Harriet Crawford,
and
Heather O'Maonaigh
with oversight from the
Committee to Study the Mortality of Military Personnel Present at Atmospheric Tests of Nuclear Weapons

NATIONAL ACADEMY PRESS
Washington, D.C.

NATIONAL ACADEMY PRESS 2101 Constitution Avenue, N.W. Washington, DC 20418

NOTICE: The project that is the subject of this report was approved by the Governing Board of the National Research Council, whose members are drawn from the councils of the National Academy of Sciences, the National Academy of Engineering, and the Institute of Medicine. The members of the advisory committee for the report were chosen for their special competences and with regard for appropriate balance.

Support for this project was provided by the Defense Threat Reduction Agency, formerly the Defense Nuclear Agency (DNA), under Contract No. DNA001-92-C-0042. The views, opinions, and/or findings contained in this report are those of the authors and should not be construed as an official Defense Threat Reduction Agency position, policy, or decision unless so designated by other documentation.

International Standard Book Number 0-309-06781-2

Additional copies of this report are available for sale from the National Academy Press , 2101 Constitution Avenue, N.W., Box 285, Washington, DC 20055. Call (800) 624-6242 or (202) 334-3313 in the Washington metropolitan area), or visit the NAP online bookstore at **www.nap.edu** .

For more information about the Institute of Medicine, visit the IOM home page at: **www.iom.edu.**

Printed in the United States of America

The serpent has been a symbol of long life, healing, and knowledge among almost all cultures and religions since the beginning of recorded history. The serpent adopted as a logotype by the Institute of Medicine is a relief carving from ancient Greece, now held by the Staatliche Museen in Berlin.

THE NATIONAL ACADEMIES

National Academy of Sciences
National Academy of Engineering
Institute of Medicine
National Research Council

The **National Academy of Sciences** is a private, nonprofit, self-perpetuating society of distinguished scholars engaged in scientific and engineering research, dedicated to the furtherance of science and technology and to their use for the general welfare. Upon the authority of the charter granted to it by the Congress in 1863, the Academy has a mandate that requires it to advise the federal government on scientific and technical matters. Dr. Bruce M. Alberts is president of the National Academy of Sciences.

The **National Academy of Engineering** was established in 1964, under the charter of the National Academy of Sciences, as a parallel organization of outstanding engineers. It is autonomous in its administration and in the selection of its members, sharing with the National Academy of Sciences the responsibility for advising the federal government. The National Academy of Engineering also sponsors engineering programs aimed at meeting national needs, encourages education and research, and recognizes the superior achievements of engineers. Dr. William A. Wulf is president of the National Academy of Engineering.

The **Institute of Medicine** was established in 1970 by the National Academy of Sciences to secure the services of eminent members of appropriate professions in the examination of policy matters pertaining to the health of the public. The Institute acts under the responsibility given to the National Academy of Sciences by its congressional charter to be an adviser to the federal government and, upon its own initiative, to identify issues of medical care, research, and education. Dr. Kenneth I. Shine is president of the Institute of Medicine.

The **National Research Council** was organized by the National Academy of Sciences in 1916 to associate the broad community of science and technology with the Academy's purposes of furthering knowledge and advising the federal government. Functioning in accordance with general policies determined by the Academy, the Council has become the principal operating agency of both the National Academy of Sciences and the National Academy of Engineering in providing services to the government, the public, and the scientific and engineering communities. The Council is administered jointly by both Academies and the Institute of Medicine. Dr. Bruce M. Alberts and Dr. William A. Wulf are chairman and vice chairman, respectively, of the National Research Council.

www.national-academies.org

AUTHORS, INSTITUTE OF MEDICINE

SUSAN THAUL (*Study Director*), Epidemiologist
WILLIAM F. PAGE, Statistician
HARRIET CRAWFORD, Operations Director
HEATHER O'MAONAIGH, Research Associate

ADVISORY COMMITTEE TO STUDY THE MORTALITY OF MILITARY PERSONNEL PRESENT AT ATMOSPHERIC TESTS OF NUCLEAR WEAPONS

Current Advisory Committee

HARVEY CHECKOWAY (*Chair*), Professor, Departments of Environmental Health and Epidemiology, University of Washington, Seattle
RICHARD J. M. FRY, Consultant, Biology Division, Oak Ridge National Laboratory, Oak Ridge, Tennessee
SAMUEL HELLMAN, A.N. Pritzker Distinguished Service Professor, Department of Radiation and Cellular Oncology, The University of Chicago
ELAINE RON, Chief, Radiation Epidemiology Branch, National Cancer Institute, National Institutes of Health, Bethesda, Maryland
WILLIAM G. SEIBERT, Senior Archivist, National Personnel Records Center, St. Louis, Missouri
JOHN E. TILL, President, Risk Assessment Corporation, Neeses, South Carolina
CLARICE R. WEINBERG, Chief, Biostatistics Branch, National Institute of Environmental Health Sciences, National Institutes of Health, Research Triangle Park, North Carolina

Former Members of Advisory Committee

CLARK W. HEATH, JR. (until 2/15/99)
DAVID HOEL (until 12/1/94)
JOHN LITTLE (until 3/9/94)
RODNEY WITHERS (until 8/9/94)

WORKING GROUP ON DOSIMETRY

JOHN E. TILL (*Chair*), committee member
F. OWEN HOFFMAN,* SENES of Oak Ridge, Inc.
KEITH J. SCHIAGER,* Department of Radiological Health, University of Utah, Salt Lake City
JOHN TASCHNER,* Los Alamos National Laboratory, New Mexico
CLARICE R. WEINBERG, committee member

MEDICAL FOLLOW-UP AGENCY

RICHARD N. MILLER, Director
PAMELA RAMEY-MCCRAY, Administrative Assistant

---

*Not a member of the advisory committee.

REVIEWERS

This report has been reviewed in draft form by individuals chosen for their diverse perspectives and technical expertise, in accordance with procedures approved by the National Research Council's Report Review Committee. The purpose of this independent review is to provide candid and critical comments that will assist the Institute of Medicine in making the published report as sound as possible and to ensure that the report meets institutional standards for objectivity, evidence, and responsiveness to the study charge. The review comments and draft manuscript remain confidential to protect the integrity of the deliberative process. The committee wishes to thank the following individuals for their participation in the review of this report:

JOHN D. BOICE, JR., International Epidemiology Institute, Rockville, Maryland

DAVID BRENNER, Center for Radiological Research, Columbia University School of Public Health, New York

ETHEL S. GILBERT, Radiation Epidemiology Branch, National Cancer Institute, National Institutes of Health, Bethesda, Maryland

MAUREEN M. HENDERSON, Department of Epidemiology, University of Washington, Seattle

MATTHEW PUGLISI, The American Legion, Washington, D.C.

JONATHAN M. SAMET, Department of Epidemiology, Johns Hopkins University School of Hygiene and Public Health, Baltimore, Maryland

RICHARD B. SETLOW, Brookhaven National Laboratory, Upton, New York

Although the individuals listed above have provided constructive comments and suggestions, it must be emphasized that responsibility for the final content of this report rests entirely with the authors and the Institute of Medicine.

Preface

For more than half a century, veterans, scientists, and the public have debated and searched for answers about whether military personnel involved in nuclear tests experienced adverse health effects because of their participation. The study we report here is the latest attempt to quantify and understand the aftermath of those tests.

Throughout the Five Series Study, the Medical Follow-up Agency staff has relied on the guidance of the Institute of Medicine advisory committee created to oversee the study. Members included leading experts in radiation and cancer epidemiology, biostatistics, radiation biology and medicine, radiation physics and dosimetry, and national archival sources. The committee provided information, leads, insight, and technical assistance and the report is better for that interaction, but responsibility for the final product rests with the staff.

This report presents the information that we could derive from this study. How scientists, the government, veterans, and the general public interpret and use that information is now open for discussion but not within the scope of this study.

Susan Thaul, Ph.D.
William F. Page, Ph.D.
Harriet Crawford, B.S.
Heather O'Maonaigh, M.A.

Acknowledgments

The study of the five series participants has been underway in some form or another since 1982. The list of people who deserve recognition for their contributions is enormous. The initial study team that began the current Five Series Study was led by Dennis Robinette, a radiation biologist who died shortly before the contract to do this study was signed. His earlier report, coauthored with Seymour Jablon and Thomas Preston, set the stage for this study.

Members of the data operations staff who worked through almost the entire life of the study were Chiquita "Squeaky" Benson, Mary Juman, and Sylvia McGinnis, joined in recent years by Jihad Daghmash. Others who worked on the data collection and management for this project include Phillip Bailey, Noah Dropkin, Nicholas Findlay, Faye Lucas, Jean Philemond, Elaine Pickens, Alex Saenger, and Denise Tyner-Parker. Erin Bell, Christopher Howson, Philip Renzullo, and Youn Shim each worked on the epidemiology of this study. Christopher Johnson, to whom this report is dedicated, was the project director and source of radiation and health physics and military radiation safety operations information for the most of the study period.

The data collection efforts for the Five Series Study involved a cast of hundreds. We appreciate the efforts of Robert Bilgrad and staff at the National Death Index; Clifford Amsler, Barbara Bauman, and staff at the National Personnel Records Center in St. Louis, Missouri; and staff at many federal archives centers and VA regional offices across the country, especially the VA regional office in the District of Columbia.

We relied on a few consultants external to the staff for some technical work critical to the conduct of the study: Charles Alcorn, Gary Marsh, Jeanette Peterson, Florence Poillon, Karl Wise, and Ada Youk. Jeremy Yu assisted during a summer internship.

The MFUA staff has benefited from the vigilance and enthusiasm of many interested veterans, especially Pat Broudy; Boley Caldwell, who provided the NAAV medical survey data used in participant validation; Robert Campbell; and Oscar Rosen.

The current members of the advisory committee to the Five Series Study— chair Harvey Checkoway, Richard J.M. Fry, Samuel Hellman, Elaine Ron, William Seibert, John Till, and Clarice Weinberg—have helped to ensure the quality of the logic followed in the conduct of this study. We thank them and assume responsibility for whatever items of advice they offered that we did not take. The committee's report to the sponsor concerning the utility for this study of the Nuclear Test Personnel Review program dose data dosimetry included contributions from invited experts not members of the committee: F. Owen Hoffman, Keith Schiager, and John Taschner. Clark Heath, Jr., David Hoel, John Little, and Rodney Withers each served as members of the advisory committee, though not to study completion.

D. Michael Schaeffer has been able to convey urgency and patience simultaneously in managing the Defense Threat Reduction Agency contract with the Institute of Medicine for this project. We thank him, Joan Ma Pierre, and the DTRA staff and contractor team, including Paul Chase and Hilda Maier of JAYCOR and Jeff Klemm of SAIC.

Sue Barron, Claudia Carl, Andrea Cohen, Mike Edington, Cheryl Greenhouse, James Jensen, Linda Kilroy, Sandra McDermin, Barbara Rice, Catherine Stryker, Kirsten Sampson Snyder, Neil Tickner, and the many other staff at the Institute of Medicine or the National Research Council all helped along the way. Special thanks to Medical Follow-up Agency director Richard Miller and administrative assistant Pamela Ramey-McCray who provided much appreciated support to the project.

We—Susan Thaul, William Page, Harriet Crawford, and Heather O'Maonaigh—thank everyone on this list (and perhaps a few whose names we have unintentionally omitted) for producing with us this Five Series Study report.

Abbreviations, Acronyms, and Glossary

a priori.	A hypothesis held prior to the conduct of analysis.
AEC.	Atomic Energy Commission.
all-cancer mortality.	All deaths attributed to any malignant neoplasm.
all-cause mortality.	All deaths.
annual dose limit.	Maximum radiation dose allowed on an annual basis.
ascertainment.	Completeness of discovery.
associated causes of death.	Conditions noted on the death certificate as contributing to an individual's death but not noted as its underlying cause.
association.	An observed relationship between variables; not necessarily indicative of causation.
atmospheric testing.	Detonating a nuclear weapon or device in the atmosphere or close to the earth's surface as part of the testing program. U.S. testing was carried out by the Atomic Energy Commission (AEC) and supported by the Department of Defense from 1945 to 1962 (JAYCOR, 1997).
atomic bomb.	A term sometimes applied to a nuclear weapon using fission energy only (Bruce-Henderson, 1982).
atomic veteran.	Veteran of the armed forces (here, Army, Navy, Air Force, or Marine Corps) present at one or more nuclear weapons tests.
badged dose.	An estimate of an individual's radiation dose as derived from one or more film badges assigned to the individual at the time of exposure.
BEIR.	Biological Effects of Ionizing Radiation; a series of reports by committees of the National Research Council, National Academy of Sciences.
BEIR V.	Fifth report on the Biological Effects of Ionizing Radiation (National Research Council, 1990).
bias.	Systematic deviation of results or inferences from the truth, or the processes leading to such deviation (Last, 1995).

BIRLS. Beneficiary Identification and Records Locator Subsystem, Department of Veterans Affairs. Electronic file of all claims; begun in 1972.

branch of service. Branch of the U.S. armed forces of which an individual was a member at the time of nuclear weapons test participation.

by-products. A secondary result, here pertaining to a nuclear reaction.

cancer. A malignant tumor.

CASTLE. Military code name of atmospheric test of nuclear weapons, 1954, Bikini and Enewetak Atolls, Marshall Islands, Pacific Proving Ground.

causal judgment. Process used to weigh pieces of evidence—including strength of association, consistency across studies, statistical significance, biologic coherence—in judging whether one event or condition might be the cause of an observed outcome.

cause of death. Condition indicated on an individual's death certificate as the underlying cause of death.

CDC. Centers for Disease Control and Prevention, DHHS.

censoring. Loss or removal of subjects from a study; observations with unknown values from one end of a frequency distribution, occurring beyond a measurement threshold (Last, 1995).

CFR. See *Code of Federal Regulations.*

chi-square (X^2) tests. Tests of statistical significance used to assess the likelihood that an observed bivariate relationship differs significantly from that which easily could have occurred by chance (Singleton et al., 1993).

CI. See *confidence interval.*

claims folder. Department of Veterans Affairs administrative paper record containing information to document the process of a veteran's claim for benefits; maintained in the VA regional office covering the geographic region of the claimant; record is retired to a federal archive records center.

CLL. Chronic lymphoid leukemia, a form of leukemia that has not been found in studies to be radiogenic. Also called chronic *lymphocytic* leukemia.

CNS. Central nervous system.

Code of Federal Regulations (CFR). A codification of the general and permanent rules published in the *Federal Register* by the executive departments and agencies of the federal government, online and as paper editions via the Government Printing Office.

cohort. A group of persons defined by a shared experience, such as an exposure.

cohort study. An epidemiologic investigation involving the follow-up of one or more groups of individuals who are known to have had an exposure or a disease and whose health status is followed over time. Can usually provide a basis for calculating risk or disease outcome.

comparison group. A group selected to have specific characteristics in common with the study group, but which has not experienced the exposure of interest.

confidence interval (CI). Used in epidemiology/statistics. States the lower and upper bounds of the statistical precision of an estimate.

confounder. A variable that is associated with the outcome under study and with exposure in the study population, but is which not a consequence of this exposure.

covariate adjustment. A process by which a statistical estimate is calculated so that the effects of other covarying factors (covariates) have been accounted for.

Cox proportional hazard ratio analysis. A statistical model in survival analysis asserting that the effect of the study factors on the risk of occurrence of an event in the study population is multiplicative and does not change over time (Last, 1995).

CROSSROADS. Military code name of atmospheric test of nuclear weapons, 1946, Bikini Atoll, Marshall Islands.

crude death rate. A measure of the proportion of the population that dies within a specified period (Last, 1995). The number of deaths in the population divided by the total population. Called "crude" because it does not adjust for age or other characteristics of the population.

custom dose estimates. An individual-level dose reconstruction.

database. An organized set of data or collection of files that can be used for a specified purpose (Last, 1995).

death certificate. A vital statistics record signed by a licensed physician or by another designated health worker that includes cause of death, decedent's name, sex, birth date, places of residence and of death, and whether the deceased had been medically attended before death (Last, 1995). Maintained by each state.

deck logs. The documents that record the daily activities of Navy and Coast Guard ships, including a listing of officers on board (JAYCOR, 1995).

Defense Nuclear Agency (DNA). The name was changed to Defense Special Weapons Agency (DSWA) in 1996 and to Defense Threat Reduction Agency (DTRA) in 1998.

Defense Special Weapons Agency (DSWA). New name for DNA as of 1996; changed to Defense Threat Reduction Agency (DTRA) in 1998.

Defense Threat Reduction Agency (DTRA). New name for DSWA as of 1998; earlier names were Defense Special Weapons Agency and Defense Nuclear Agency.

descriptive analyses. Quantitative comparisons designed to describe the existing distribution of variables without immediate regard to cause or other hypotheses.

deterministic effects. Acute radiation effects, often due to cell killing; for example, burns and nausea.

DHHS. Department of Health and Human Services, U.S.

diagnosis codes. International Classification of Disease codes that associate a unique code number to standard cause-of-death definitions.

diagnostic radiology.	The medical use of radiation as a means of investigating and diagnosing disease.
differential.	Showing a difference, usually used in a context where a difference can produce bias.
discrepancy.	Disagreement or divergence between facts or claims.
DNA.	See *Defense Nuclear Agency.*
DoD.	Department of Defense, U.S.
dose.	A measurement of the biological effect of radiation on the human body; referred to as dose equivalent and measured in sievert (rem) (JAYCOR, 1997).
dose reconstruction.	A scientific analysis of the radiological aspects of an environment in space and time, used to calculate radiation levels from which an estimate of dose is made of the dose to an individual in that environment (JAYCOR, 1997).
dosimetry.	The measurement and recording of radiation doses and dose rates (Bruce-Henderson, 1982). As used in the NTPR program, this term applies only to doses obtained from dosimeters (JAYCOR, 1997).
Dose–response relationship.	A relationship in which a change in amount, intensity, or duration of exposure is associated with a change in the rate or amount of a specific outcome (Last, 1995).
DSWA.	See *Defense Special Weapons Agency.*
DTRA.	See *Defense Threat Reduction Agency.*
E1–E7.	Enlisted personnel paygrades.
elevated risk.	Risk that is elevated relative to that observed in a comparison population.
endpoints.	Outcomes. Here, death or death due to a specific cause.
Enewetak.	Atoll in the northwestern Marshall Islands in the Pacific Ocean.
epidemiology.	The study of the distribution and determinants of health-related states or events in specified populations, and the application of this study to the control health problems (Last, 1995).
estimate.	A measure or statement about the value of some quantity that is said to be an estimate if it is known, believed, or suspected to incorporate some degree of error (Last, 1995).
excess mortality.	The amount by which the number of deaths observed in a group exceeds the number expected absent the exposure of interest.
expected mortality.	A baseline standard of mortality that would be expected absent the exposure under study; can be calculated from standard population rates or from an unexposed comparison population.
exposure (radiation).	A term describing the amount of ionizing radiation that is incident upon living or inanimate material.
exposure surrogates.	Proxy measures used in instances in which the actual exposure of interest cannot be reliably assessed.

fact of death.	Ascertainment of vital status (whether an individual is alive or dead) without respect to cause.
fallout.	Material (mostly radioactive) lofted into a nuclear cloud and later deposited over an area (JAYCOR, 1997).
FARC.	Federal archives records center; repository of retired government records such as VA claims folders.
film badge.	Photographic film shielded from light and worn by an individual to measure and record radiation dose.
follow-on studies.	Future research endeavors warranted or proposed based on study results.
follow-up period.	The period of time during which observations are made of an individual, group, or initially defined population whose appropriate characteristics have been assessed in order to observe changes in health status or health-related variables (Last, 1995).
GAO.	See *General Accounting Office.*
General Accounting Office (GAO).	The General Accounting Office is the investigative arm of Congress. Charged with examining matters relating to the receipt and disbursement of public funds, GAO performs audits and evaluations of government programs and activities.
grade.	A classification of military rank into categories.
GREENHOUSE.	Military code name of atmospheric test of nuclear weapons, 1951, Enewetak Atoll, Marshall Islands.
ground zero.	The point on the surface of land or water at, or vertically below or above, the center of the burst of a nuclear weapon (Bruce-Henderson, 1982).
hazard ratio (HR).	The probability of the occurrence of an event for an individual in a study population divided by the probability of the occurrence of an event in a comparison population.
HCFA.	Health Care Financing Administration, DHHS.
healthy soldier effect.	The observed tendency of soldiers, as an aggregated group, to be in better health than the general United States population because of pre-induction selection and continuing military health and performance standards.
healthy worker effect.	The observed tendency of workers, as an aggregated group, to be in better health than the general United States population.
hematologic cancers.	Cancers of the blood-forming organs, including the leukemias, Hodgkin's disease, non-Hodgkin's lymphoma, and other lymphopoietic cancers.
HR.	See *hazard ratio.*
ICD9.	*International Classification of Diseases,* 9th revision. (See References: USDHHS, 1991)
ICRP.	International Commission on Radiological Protection.

incidence.	The number of persons who have developed a disease in a given period of time divided by the total population at risk.
IOM.	Institute of Medicine.
ionizing radiation.	Radiation that produces ion pairs along its path through a substance.
JAYCOR.	A company providing contract services to the Defense Threat Reduction Agency; involved with the Nuclear Test Personnel Review program.
kiloton (kt).	1,000 tons.
known dead.	Identified as deceased as the result of records investigation.
kt.	See *kiloton.*
land series.	For this report, a nuclear weapons test series occurring at the Nevada Test Site (NTS) in the continental United States. In this report, Operations UPSHOT-KNOTHOLE and PLUMBBOB.
latency period.	Delay between exposure to a disease-causing agent and the appearance or manifestation of the disease (Last, 1995).
leukemia.	Any of several types of cancer in which there is usually a disorganized proliferation of white blood cells in the bone marrow (AMA, 1989).
Life Span Study (LSS).	Ongoing follow-up of the population exposed to atomic bomb detonations in Hiroshima and Nagasaki, Japan, and progeny; conducted by the Radiation Effects Research Foundation.
LSS.	See *Life Span Study.*
malignancy.	See *malignant neoplasm.*
malignant neoplasm.	A tumor (neoplasm) that spreads from its site of origin to affect other parts of the body.
matched.	Chosen for comparison based on selected shared characteristics.
mathematical model.	A representation of a system, process, or relationship in mathematical form in which equations are used to estimate the behavior of the system or the process under study (Last, 1995).
megaton (Mt).	1 million tons. Here, the explosive energy equivalent to 1,000,000 metric tons of TNT.
MFUA.	Medical Follow-up Agency, Institute of Medicine.
military unit.	Organized body of military personnel which may contain only a few, or as many as thousands of members (JAYCOR, 1995).
millirem (mrem).	One-thousandth of a rem; equivalent to 0.01 mSv.
millisievert (mSv).	One-thousandth of a sievert; equivalent to 100 mrem.
morbidity.	Any departure, subjective or objective, from a state of physiological or psychological well-being (Last, 1995). Illness.
morning reports.	Documents maintained by the Army and Air Force to recordthe daily duty status changes, such as arrivals, departures, absences, ill

	nesses, etc. of personnel assigned to company/battery/squadron and headquarters level units (JAYCOR, 1995).
mortality.	Death.
mrem.	See *millirem.*
MSN.	Military service number; identification number used for military service personnel.
mSv.	See *millisievert.*
Mt.	See *megaton.*
muster rolls.	Documents that record the assignment of Navy and Coast Guard enlisted personnel aboard ships (JAYCOR, 1995).
NAAV.	National Association of Atomic Veterans.
NARA.	National Archives and Records Administration.
NAS.	National Academy of Sciences; component of the National Academies.
National Center for Health Statistics (NCHS).	Part of the Centers for Disease Control and Prevention; maintains the National Death Index.
National Death Index (NDI).	Maintained by the National Center for Health Statistics, CDC, DHHS; compiles death certificate information since 1979 from all U.S. states, the District of Columbia, and New York City, as well as territories and protectorates; provides name of state in which death occurred and death certificate number to researchers (following extensive institutional review board procedures).
natural background radiation.	Ionizing radiation encountered in everyday life, primarily from terrestrial radioactivity (e.g., radon) and cosmic rays. Approximately 3 mSv per year for persons living in the United States.
NCHS.	National Center for Health Statistics.
NCRP.	National Council on Radiation Protection and Measurements.
NDI.	See *National Death Index.*
NDI-Plus.	Recently added NDI service; provides to researchers coded and computerized causes of death (so researcher need not contact each state individually).
nested case-control study.	A case-control study (study of individuals with an outcome of interest relative to a suitable comparison group) conducted within a subset of an entire cohort.
Nevada Test Site (NTS).	The region in Nevada set aside for the continental atmospheric nuclear weapons testing program. Also referred to as the Nevada Proving Ground (NPG) (Gladeck and Johnson, 1996).
nonparticipants.	Individuals included in the study specifically identified as not having participated in any nuclear weapons testing or in the bombing or occupation of Hiroshima and Nagasaki, Japan; nor having been a prisoner of war in Japan at the time of the bombing. In this report, nonparticipants are also called referents and members of the referent cohort.
nosologist.	An individual trained in the classification of diagnoses as recorded in medical records or death certificates according to established categories.
not known dead.	Not identified as deceased following records investigation.

NPRC.	National Personnel Records Center, St. Louis, Missouri.
NRC.	National Research Council; a component of the National Academies.
NRPB.	National Radiological Protection Board, U.K.
NTPR.	See *Nuclear Test Personnel Review Program.*
NTS.	See *Nevada Test Site.*
nuclear device.	Any device in which the explosion results from the energy released by reaction involving atomic nuclei (Bruce-Henderson, 1982).
Nuclear Regulatory Commission.	Independent regulatory agency established by the U.S. Congress to ensure adequate protection of the public health and safety, the common defense and security, and the environment in the use of nuclear materials in the United States.
Nuclear Test Personnel Review (NTPR) Program.	Maintained by the Defense Threat Reduction Agency, DoD.
nuclear weapon.	See *nuclear device* (Bruce-Henderson, 1982).
O1–O10.	Commissioned officer paygrades.
observed to expected.	Comparison of number of observed events (e.g., deaths) in one group with expected values based on a standard or specifically chosen comparison population.
OCMAP; OCMAP-PLUS.	Occupational Cohort Mortality Analysis Program. Computer program developed by Gary Marsh and others at the University of Pittsburgh Department of Biostatistics.
Office of Technology Assessment (OTA).	Former nonpartisan research unit within the U.S. Congress that provided congressional committees analyses of emerging, difficult, and often highly technical issues and helped to identify policy options.
OTA.	See *Office of Technology Assessment.*
outcome measures.	Measures of the possible results that may stem from an exposure to a causal factor (Last, 1995).
oversight committee.	A National Research Council volunteer committee of experts that provides guidance, but does not author a report.
p.	Probability (epidemiology/statistics, e.g., $p = .05$). See Appendix C.
Pacific Proving Ground (PPG).	Site of most U.S. oceanic nuclear weapons tests. Consisted primarily of the Enewetak and Bikini Atolls in the north-western Marshall Islands of the Pacific Ocean (Gladeck and Johnson, 1996).
participating unit.	Military unit designations by which individuals are associated with an atmospheric nuclear test. These are the units that members participated with during the test (JAYCOR, 1995).
paygrade.	Referred to in military records as a *payrate,* it is uniform across the branches of service; examples are E3 (third grade enlisted personnel 3) and O1 (lowest grade officer).

permanent unit. Military units that participants were permanently assigned to during the operation. It was common for a veteran's permanent unit and participating unit to be the same (JAYCOR, 1995).

personal dosimeters. Devices (usually film badges) for measuring radiation dose to an individual.

personnel roster. Air Force, Army, and Marine Corps documents that list the name, military service number, and grade or rank or rate of each person in a unit on a given date.

PHREG. Proportional hazards regression program, SAS.

PLUMBBOB. Military code name of atmospheric test of nuclear weapons, 1957, Nevada Test Site.

potential radiation exposure. Radiation exposures of uncertain occurrence.

PPG. See *Pacific Proving Ground.*

radiation. Energy propagated through space or matter as waves (gamma rays, ultraviolet light) or as particles (alpha or beta rays). External radiation is from a source outside the body, whereas internal radiation is from a source inside the body (e.g., radionuclides deposited in tissues).

Radiation Effects Research Foundation (RERF). A cooperative Japan-United States research organization.

radiogenic. Causally linked to radiation.

RADSAFE. Military units or personnel that provide radiation safety monitoring functions.

rank. Personnel grades—sometimes referred to as *ratings;* examples include Admiral, General, Private, and Seaman (JAYCOR, 1995); these are not consistent across branches of service.

ratio. The value obtained by dividing one quantity by another (Last, 1995).

REDWING. Military code name of atmospheric test of nuclear weapons, 1956, Bikini and Enewetak Atolls, Marshall Islands.

referent. Member of a comparison group or the comparison group itself.

referent population. The standard against which a population being studied can be compared.

regression. Statistical analysis that seeks to determine the "best" mathematical function to describe a series of data points.

relative risk (RR). The ratio of the incidence of a condition in the exposed population divided by the incidence in the nonexposed population. If there is no difference as a result of exposure, the RR is 1.0.

rem. A unit of radiation dose equivalent; replaced by the sievert; 1 rem is equivalent to 0.01 Sv.

RERF. See *Radiation Effects Research Foundation.*

risk. The probability that an event will occur.

RR. See *relative risk.*

SAS. Originally "Statistical Analysis System," proprietary software package.

sea series. Oceanic nuclear weapons test series. In this report, Operations GREENHOUSE, CASTLE, AND REDWING.

selection series. For this study, the first (or only) of the five studied series in which a member of the participant cohort was present; the selection series for a member of the referent cohort is the series corresponding to the time period and set of unit matching criteria that was used to select the participant cohort.

series. An official grouping of nuclear weapons tests.

shield (shielding). A body of material used to physically reduce the intensity of radiation.

shot. The detonation of a nuclear device; used synonymously with *test* in discussion of the atmospheric nuclear weapons testing program.

SI. International System of Units (as instituted in 1960).

sievert (Sv). A unit of effective or equivalent dose. Equivalent dose incorporates an adjustment for the fact that different types of radiation (alpha, beta, gamma, neutron) differ in their ability to do biologic damage. Effective dose also incorporates adjustments for the relative sensitivity of different organ systems. The sievert is the SI unit that replaced the rem. 1 Sv is equivalent to 100 rem.

SMR. Standardized mortality ratio. See Chapter 9.

SSN. Social Security number.

statistical adjustment. The use of statistical methods to control for potentially biasing factors in an analysis.

statistical significance. See Appendix C.

stratification. The process of or result of separating a sample into several sub-samples according to specified criteria (e.g., age, sex) (Last, 1995).

survival time. The period of study time that an individual is observed until the occurrence of the outcome of interest or the end of the study.

Sv. See *sievert.*

systematic differences. Differences that are not randomly distributed.

tests. The detonation of a nuclear weapon (device); also called a *shot.*

thermonuclear device. Fusion-based nuclear weapons.

time-dependent. Not constant over time.

timescale. Units selected for the measurement of time, for example, calendar time or age.

tumor. An abnormal mass of tissue that forms when cells in a specific area reproduce at an increased rate. Also known as a neoplasm. May benign or malignant (AMA, 1989).

underlying cause of death. The disease or injury that initiated the train of events leading to death or the circumstances of the accident of violence that produced fatal injury (Last, 1995).

unit diary. The document that recorded the daily duty status changes personnel assigned to Marine Corps company-level units (JAYCOR, 1995).

United Nations Scientific Committee on the Effects of Atomic Radiation (UNSCEAR). A committee of the U.N. General Assembly.

UNSCEAR.	See *United Nations Scientific Committee on the Effects of Atomic Radiation.*
UPSHOT-KNOTHOLE.	Military code name of atmospheric test of nuclear weapons, 1953, Nevada Test Site.
US.	United States.
USS.	United States Ship, Navy.
VA.	Department of Veterans Affairs.
validation.	Exercise to assess acceptability of data ascertainment.
VAMI.	See *Veterans Administration Master Index.*
VARO.	Veterans Affairs regional office.
verification.	Efforts to verify that information obtained is accurate.
Veterans Administration Master Index (VAMI).	Index cards for each VA beneficiary; system superseded by BIRLS in 1972.
vital status.	Determination as to whether an individual is alive or deceased.
W1–W4.	Warrant officer paygrades.
yield.	The total effective energy released in a nuclear detonation (Gladeck and Johnson, 1996).

Contents

TABLES

DEDICATION

We dedicate this report to J. Christopher Johnson
(1949–1999)

Summary

More than 200,000 U.S. military personnel participated in atmospheric nuclear weapons tests between 1945 and the 1963 Limited Nuclear Test Ban Treaty. Questions persist, such as whether that test participation is associated with the timing and causes of death among those individuals. This is the report of a mortality study of the approximately 70,000 soldiers, sailors, and airmen who participated in at least one of five selected U.S. nuclear weapons test series[1] in the 1950s and nearly 65,000 comparable nonparticipants, the referents. The investigation described in this report, based on more than 5 million person-years of mortality follow-up, represents one of the largest cohort studies of military veterans ever conducted. We found that, during the follow-up period,

- overall, participants and referents had similar risks of death;
- participants and referents had similar risks of death from cancer; and
- specifically, participants had an apparent 14 percent higher risk of leukemia death than the referents, although that difference was not statistically significant and could be a chance finding.

Descriptive analyses not specified at the outset of this study showed

- statistically significant increased risk of leukemia death among participants at land test series (tests conducted at the Nevada Test Site) compared to land series referents; however, sea series participants (tests conducted at the Pa

[1] Series selected were Operations GREENHOUSE (1951), UPSHOT-KNOTHOLE (1953), CASTLE (1954), REDWING (1956), and PLUMBBOB (1957). These five series were chosen for an earlier study of atomic veterans to represent tests at both the Nevada Test Site and the Pacific Proving Ground. Fuller discussion is in Chapter 1.

cific Proving Ground) have an observed and not significant lower risk than sea series referents;

- statistically significant increased risk of all-cause mortality among participants at sea series (tests conducted at the Pacific Proving Ground) compared to sea series referents; and
- statistically significant increased risks among participants of death from external causes (such as motor vehicle accidents), nasal cancer, and prostate cancer.

The leukemia findings do not resolve the debate over whether either participation in general or the radiation doses in particular is associated with leukemia mortality. The set of leukemia findings is consistent with the results of other studies of military participants in nuclear tests and is consistent with a hypothesis that these are radiation effects. The other findings listed are more likely to be chance occurrences. We discuss the evidence in greater detail in the report.

METHODS

The participant cohort—predominantly white and male—was identified from the database maintained by the Nuclear Test Personnel Review Program (NTPR) at the Defense Threat Reduction Agency.[2] This study supersedes an earlier National Research Council report (Robinette et al., 1985) that was based on a different NTPR-provided dataset that was subsequently identified as inaccurate.[3] The Medical Follow-up Agency (MFUA) and NTPR staff have placed substantial effort into validating the current participation list. We verified that the individuals it includes were indeed participants in these test series and we estimated that the list might have missed approximately one percent of actual participants.

We compared the participant cohort's mortality experience with that of a referent cohort of military personnel comparable to the participants with respect to branch of service, time of active military duty, type and general location of assigned unit, age, and paygrade. Department of Veterans Affairs (VA) records and databases provided fact of death for members of both cohorts. For each identified death, cause of death information was requested from VA regional offices and federal archives records centers, where VA claims folders, which hold death certificates, are filed. In those cases for which cause of death was not available through that route, we searched the database of the National Death Index for death certificate-derived cause of death information.

---

[2] The organizational locus of the Nuclear Test Personnel Review Program within the Department of Defense was the Defense Nuclear Agency, renamed the Defense Special Weapons Agency in June 1996, and reorganized in October 1998 as the Defense Threat Reduction Agency.

[3] Chapter 1 of the full report describes the history in greater detail.

Using two analytic techniques—proportional hazards models and standardized mortality ratios—we tested for differences between the participant and referent cohorts in all-cause, all-cancer, and leukemia mortality. Analyses based on the proportional hazards model involve direct comparisons of the participant and referent cohorts, whereas standardized mortality ratios involve comparison of each group, separately, with external population rates. Further explorations included other outcomes (e.g., all major categories of deaths, and specific groupings of cancers) and possible differences in effect for participants of test series conducted at the Pacific Proving Ground (sea series) and participants at the Nevada Test Site (land series).

The initial plan for this epidemiologic study included the use of individual-level radiation dose data, compiled and estimated by NTPR, to test for dose-response relationships indicative of radiation-caused adverse health effects. However, the Institute of Medicine committee overseeing the conduct of this study reviewed the dosimetry program and found that the dose data were not appropriate for epidemiologic analysis. Thus, no dose data were used in analyses for this report. The committee's letter report to the Defense Nuclear Agency, this study's sponsor and the Department of Defense entity responsible for the NTPR program, describes the relevant limitations of the data for these purposes and suggests ways to create dose data that could be appropriate for epidemiologic use (IOM, 1995; reprinted in this report as Appendix A).

FINDINGS AND DISCUSSION

Veteran concern about radiogenic cancer was a major impetus for this research. That leukemia, the cancer most consistently linked with radiation, is fairly rare is fortunate. However, that presents an obstacle to a study of this kind. Only a study cohort four times the size of the one available would have been likely to identify the observed leukemia risk as statistically significant.

Although dose data might have increased the study's statistical power to detect an increased risk among participants (if there were an increased risk), these data were judged inappropriate for epidemiologic analysis. In the absence of epidemiologically useful dose data, the focus of this research shifted to an examination of the hazards associated with test participation, irrespective of dose. Overall, no statistically significant differences are evident in all-cause, all-cancer, or leukemia mortality between participants and referents. However, although not statistically significant, the risk of leukemia mortality was elevated in participants compared to referents. Among the leukemia subtypes, the highest relative risk of death was for lymphoid leukemia, excluding chronic lymphoid leukemia. While the estimated relative risk of leukemia mortality was higher among participants in land series than among participants in sea series, there was no articulated *a priori* basis to have predicted such a finding. Also not identified *a priori* was the association between sea series participation and all-cause mortality that we observed in this study. In addition, significantly elevated rates of death due to external causes of injury, nasal cancer, and prostate cancer were found among participants, again compared to referents.

The set of leukemia findings presented here is broadly consistent with a radiogenic cause, but is not conclusive. An increase in external causes of death has been found in other studies of military personnel who were not exposed to radiation. Explanations other than radiation effects might be pursued. Other findings—nasal and prostate cancers—would not have been expected based on other studies of the health effects of radiation exposure.

What, then, is the substantive significance of these findings? We can state that the participant group *as a whole* did not experience widespread early death. Even for leukemia, for example, there were an estimated 25 excess deaths in the participant cohort. That might be a comfort to those veterans who are not sick and to their families. The report findings to do not rule out, however, possible increased risk among distinct subgroups of test participants that this study did not have the information to identify accurately.

Stronger supporting evidence could be acquired from a further study that would make use of data on radiation dose if those data could be developed. Although the oversight committee concluded that the dose data in their current form were unsuitable for epidemiologic analysis, it also concluded that carefully carried out custom dose reconstructions done anew for selected participants, using consistent methodology, could provide usable dose data. An efficient research design (to minimize the prohibitive cost of custom dose reconstructions) requiring fewer individuals is a nested case-control study, which could focus on specific endpoints of interest, such as leukemia. The pattern of radiation dose among the leukemia deaths (cases) would be contrasted to the pattern among a sampled set of participant controls to assess a hypothesized dose-response association.

The size, length of follow-up, and persistence of data collection efforts involved in this Five Series Study have helped to assure us that the findings we report are valid. It is unlikely that another cohort study of this type and magnitude would provide more precise answers than this one, because any atomic veteran study of this kind would face the same methodologic problems, namely inadequate exposure (dose) data and imperfect mortality ascertainment, encountered in this Five Series Study.

1

Study Rationale and Overview

RATIONALE

Did participation in the U.S. nuclear weapons test program harm the military personnel involved? Reported effects range from nonfatal skin and eye conditions to cancers—both incident and fatal. The epidemiologic study presented in this report addresses mortality alone. It examines whether participants died sooner than nonparticipants or were more likely to die from specific causes such as leukemia. From the results, one may deduce—but not establish—the extent to which radiation exposure may have caused the different mortality rates, if any, in the two groups. This study, however, does not address questions concerning the relationships between test participation or radiation exposure and nonfatal adverse health effects.

BACKGROUND

In 1976, a veteran asserted that his acute myelocytic leukemia was related to his participation in Shot SMOKY, a test in the 1957 Operation PLUMBBOB series at the Nevada Test Site. In response, the Centers for Disease Control (now Centers for Disease Control and Prevention) mounted an epidemiologic study of military personnel who had attended this test and found more than the expected number of leukemia cases among participants (Caldwell et al., 1980; Caldwell et al., 1983). This generated concern that participation in the atmospheric testing program may have adversely affected health.

In 1981, the Medical Follow-up Agency (MFUA) of the National Academy of Sciences designed a study to evaluate the question of increased mortality among test participants beyond those present at Shot SMOKY. MFUA researchers, working with the Defense Nuclear Agency,[1] chose to study five of the 19 U.S.-conducted atmospheric test series. These five—Operations GREENHOUSE (1951), UPSHOT-KNOTHOLE (1953), CASTLE (1954), REDWING (1956), and PLUMBBOB (1957)—represent tests at the Pacific and Nevada test sites, substantial numbers of personnel from each of the branches of military service, and different kinds of nuclear devices. In that study (Robinette et al., 1985), the mortality experience of approximately 49,000 veterans identified by the Defense Nuclear Agency (DNA) as having participated in at least one of the five selected test series was compared to mortality rates in the U.S. male population.

In 1989, the Defense Nuclear Agency (DNA) informed MFUA that the data it had provided—on which all MFUA analyses were based—incorrectly identified many members of the participant cohort. MFUA (with the support and concurrence of the congressional Office of Technology Assessment [Gelband, 1992], the General Accounting Office [GAO, 1992], members of Congress, and Department of Defense staff) decided that the published study results should be withdrawn from discussion pending correction of the possibly substantial errors in participant group identification and subsequent reexamination of the data. At the request of the DNA, MFUA has redone the Five Series Study. We present the results of that study in this report.

In addition to the essential clarification of participant cohort membership, which resulted in a substantial increase in the number of participants, the new Five Series Study also includes a referent group of military personnel who did not participate in nuclear tests, a design element that enhances its usefulness. We took advantage, also, of the additional 11 years of mortality experience that had accrued since the completion of the first study.

In July 1992, the Institute of Medicine established an eight-member committee representing expertise in epidemiology, biostatistics, radiation biology, radiation medicine, military records, and health physics to advise MFUA staff. This committee provided oversight concerning methods of exposure-data ascertainment, mortality assessment, referent group selection, radiation effects on human health, consideration of carcinogenesis mechanisms, statistical methods, and military records use. The committee was chaired for many years by Clark Heath, Jr., M.D., then vice president for epidemiology and surveillance research at the American Cancer Society. Committee member Harvey Checkoway, Ph.D., professor, Departments of Environmental Health and Epidemiology, at the University of Washington in Seattle, assumed the chair recently when Dr. Heath accepted a staff position with the Radiation Effects Research Foundation in Hiroshima, Japan (its affiliation with the National Research Council makes him ineligible to serve as a committee member).

[1] The organizational locus of the Nuclear Test Personnel Review Program within the Department of Defense has been the Defense Nuclear Agency (until June 1996), the Defense Special Weapons Agency (until October 1998), and, currently, the Defense Threat Reduction Agency.

OVERVIEW

This study addresses one main question: Did participation in at least one of the five selected nuclear weapons test series change the risk of death for the military personnel involved? We statistically compared the mortality experience of these 68,168 participant individuals with:

- a referent group of 64,781 veterans chosen to be comparable to participants with respect to age, paygrade, branch of service, time of military service, and type of assigned military unit but who were not participants in any nuclear test; and
- the U.S. white male population.

In discussing the Five Series Study findings, we compare them with the findings of studies that examined mortality among other groups of military veterans who participated in nuclear tests.

The Defense Nuclear Agency defined membership in the participant group (see Chapter 5). We constructed a referent group, beginning with a list of DNA-identified comparable military units (see Chapter 6). Using records of the Department of Veterans Affairs and the National Archives and Records Administration (see Chapter 4), we identified individuals from the participating and referent units and deaths among these individuals. Death certificates and a death certificate-derived national database were the sources of cause-of-death information (see Chapter 4 and Chapter 8). In the study's primary analyses, we examined the numbers and timing of deaths from any cause, any malignancy, and leukemia in the two groups. Additional analytic work involved the use of more detailed, though still broad, cause-of-death categories and the exploration of characteristics of the participation experience for evidence consistent with a radiation-caused effect (see Chapter 11). Initial plans to examine dose–response relationships were changed when a working group[2] formed by the study's advisory committee determined that the available dose data were inappropriate for use in individual-level epidemiologic analyses (see Chapter 7 and Appendix A).

The report contains a brief overview of other types of studies of radiation exposure and effects on human health (Chapter 2); a description of the U.S. nuclear test program in general and the five series that are the focus of this study (Chapter 3); other methodologic issues (Chapter 4, Chapter 5, Chapter 6, Chapter 7 through Chapter 8); the analysis structure (Chapter 9); description of the participant and referent cohorts (Chapter 10); the analytic findings (Chapter 11); and our discussion of these findings (Chapter 12). Appendixes contain technical detail not essential to understanding the study but of interest to some readers and useful for documentation purposes.

---

[2] John Till, Ph.D., served as chair of the dosimetry working group, which included one other oversight committee member (Clarice Weinberg, Ph.D.) and three external dosimetry experts (F. Owen Hoffman, Ph.D.; Keith J. Schiager, Ph.D.; and John Taschner).

2

Other Studies of Radiation Exposure of Military Personnel

INTRODUCTION

The purpose of this chapter is to provide some context for later discussion of results —in particular, to discuss whether the findings of our study are consistent with what is known about the effects of radiation exposure. However, because radiation exposure data have not been used in this report (see Chapter 7), and because our discussion of the effects of radiation exposure is necessarily indirect, we do not provide an extensive discussion of dose-related radiation effects in this chapter. Furthermore, there are several excellent, recent references on radiation risk which the interested reader may consult (ICRP, 1991; National Research Council, 1990; UNSCEAR, 1994). We do discuss in some detail the results of four previous mortality studies of military veterans involved in nuclear weapons tests because the types of exposures to which they may have been subjected (both radiation and nonradiation exposures) are more likely to be similar to those experienced by the five-series cohort than those of nonmilitary cohorts.

Among the studies of nonmilitary cohorts, the study of the survivor experience following the atomic bomb exposures in Hiroshima and Nagasaki—the Life Span Study (LSS)—is of great importance despite the unique circumstances surrounding these exposures; most radiation protection recommendations are based primarily on LSS risk estimates (Ron et al., 1994). The interested reader is referred to an extensive literature on cancer incidence rates and cancer mortality rates (fairly recent examples include Land, 1995; Mabuchi et al., 1994; Nagataki et al., 1994; Pierce et al., 1996; Preston et al., 1994; Ron et al., 1994; Thompson et al., 1994); Schull (1995) provided a good overview of the entire LSS program.

Other studies of nonmilitary populations exposed to relatively high levels of radiation include the following: the Ankylosing Spondylitis Treatment Study (Darby et al., 1987); the Cervical Cancer Treatment Study (Boice et al., 1988); the Canadian Fluoroscopy Study (Sherman et al., 1978); the New York State Post partum Mastitis Study (Shore et al., 1986); and the Massachusetts Fluoroscopy Study (Boice et al., 1978, 1981). The results of such studies are typically extrapolated mathematically to provide estimates of health effects at relatively low doses.

While studies of relatively low-dose exposures can provide a basis for ensuring that radiation risk estimates based on higher doses neither underestimate nor overestimate the effects of lower doses, they have their unique problems. Chief among these are low statistical power (leading to lack of precision in risk estimates) and the strong potential for confounding that is present in studies that attempt to produce estimates of low relative risks. Studies of relatively low-level radiation exposure in nonmilitary populations include studies of exposures due to diagnostic radiology; fallout from nuclear weapons testing (populations of residents downwind from test sites); occupational exposures; and natural background radiation. The results of these kinds of studies have been reviewed in detail elsewhere (Boice, 1996; Boice, et al., 1996; NRC, 1990; and Ron, 1998).

MILITARY POPULATIONS

Several epidemiologic studies of military personnel possibly exposed to radiation during atmospheric nuclear weapons testing have contributed to the scientific debate regarding the adverse effects of radiation exposure on human health. These studies have reported modest elevations in risk for all-cause, all-cancer, and leukemia mortality in participants relative to comparison groups, but these elevations have not consistently reached statistical significance. Table 2-1 displays findings from several of the larger, controlled studies of military personnel who participated in nuclear weapons testing.

Watanabe and colleagues (1995) compared the mortality experiences of some 8,550 military participants at Operation Hardtack I, a 1958 U.S. test series in the Pacific Proving Ground, with a comparison group of roughly 14,600 military personnel. All-cause mortality (crude death rate ratio [RR] 1.10; 95% confidence interval [CI] 1.02–1.19) and digestive cancer mortality (RR 1.47; CI 1.06–2.04) were higher among participants than comparisons. Mortality rates due to all cancers, leukemia, and other suspected radiogenic cancers were not significantly elevated among participants. When stratified by gamma radiation doses—the advisability of which the advisory committee of this report questions (see Appendix A)—participants in the highest dose group (>1,000 millirem [mrem]) had significant increases in mortality for all causes (RR 1.23; CI 1.04– 1.45), all cancers (RR 1.42; CI 1.03–1.96), and liver cancer (RR 6.42; CI 1.17–35.33). Participants in the middle dose group (250–1,000 mrem) did not demonstrate increased mortality rates for any conditions. Participants in the low-dose level (0–250 mrem) had significantly increased mortality rates due to digestive organ cancer. Among the digestive organs, esophageal cancer mortality showed the largest elevation in risk (RR 2.15), although neither it nor any other individually classified digestive organ reached statistical significance.

TABLE 2-1. Selected Findings from Studies of Military Participants at Atomic Tests

Cause of Death	Darby et al., 1993a,b United Kingdom 21,358 participants 22,333 comparisons SMR Ratio (90% CI)	Pearce et al., 1996, 1997 New Zealand 528 participants 1,504 comparisons SMR Ratio (90% CI)	Watanabe et al., 1995 United States (Navy) 1,094 participants 14,625 comparisons Relative Risk (95% CI) >1,000 mrem	Watanabe et al., 1995 United States (Navy) 8,554 participants 14,625 comparisons Crude Death Rate Ratio (95% CI)	Johnson et al., 1996 United States (Navy) 38,668 participants 35,036 comparisons Hazard Ratio (95% CI)
All cause	1.01 (0.95, 1.07)	1.06 (0.87, 1.30)	1.23 (1.04, 1.45)	1.10 (1.02, 1.19)	1.05 (1.02, 1.07)
Leukemia	1.75 (1.01, 3.06)[a]	5.59 (1.04, 41.7)	1.73 (0.39, 7.56)	0.69 (0.27, 1.78)	1.02 (0.75, 1.39)
All cancer	0.95 (0.87, 1.04)	1.19 (0.84, 1.67)	1.42 (1.03, 1.96)	1.14 (0.98, 1.33)	1.01 (0.96, 1.07)
All hematologic	ND[b]	3.75 (1.36, 10.8)	ND	ND	0.98 (0.82, 1.17)
All nonhematologic	ND	1.00 (0.67, 1.45)	ND	ND	ND*
All nonneoplastic	1.01 (0.75, 1.35)	1.00 (0.77, 1.29)	ND	ND	0.97 (0.59, 1.59)
All digestive cancer	ND	0.38 (0.06, 1.36)	1.39 (0.67, 2.89)	1.47 (1.06, 2.04)	1.02 (0.91, 1.14)
Esophagus	1.19 (0.79, 1.80)	2.83 (0.31, 26.20)	—	1.16 (0.52, 2.58)	1.17 (0.87, 1.57)
Stomach	0.94 (0.66, 1.32)	0.28 (0.01, 1.60)	—	0.58 (0.19, 1.80)	1.04 (0.78, 1.38)
Large intestine (colon)	ND	0.80 (0.12, 3.44)	0.99 (0.24, 4.19)	1.28 (0.72, 2.28)	0.93 (0.77, 1.13)

Large intestine (rectum)	1.04 (0.79, 1.36)	0.56 (0.02, 3.91)	ND	ND	0.84 (0.57, 1.28)
Liver	2.46 (0.92, 6.92)	ND	6.42 (1.17, 35.33)	2.00 (0.54, 7.45)	1.49 (0.87, 2.57)
Pancreas	1.11 (0.74, 1.68)	ND	1.00 (0.13, 7.64)	1.73 (0.82, 3.63)	1.11 (0.86, 1.44)
All respiratory cancer	ND	0.92 (0.28, 2.61)	ND	1.04 (0.81, 1.34)	1.04 (0.96, 1.12)
Lung	0.85 (0.73, 0.99)	0.94 (0.45, 1.84)	1.16 (0.66, 2.05)	1.07 (0.83, 1.38)	1.05 (0.96, 1.14)
Skin[c]	1.22 (0.61, 2.44)	ND	—	0.63 (0.20, 1.98)	0.82 (0.58, 1.16)
Prostate	0.93 (0.62, 1.41)	0.35 (0.02, 2.08)	1.46 (0.34, 6.31)	1.41 (0.71, 2.80)	0.77 (0.61, 0.97)
Bladder	2.69 (1.42, 5.41)	ND	ND	0.36 (0.04, 3.08)	0.96 (0.64, 1.46)
Non-Hodgkin's	1.02 (0.55, 1.89)	5.67 (0.44, 165)	1.90 (0.23, 15.42)	1.47 (0.49, 4.37)	ND
Multiple myeloma	1.51 (0.55, 4.26)	1.41 (0.05, 18)	ND	0.54 (0.11, 2.68)	0.89 (0.55, 1.45)
Thyroid	0.00 (0.00, 13.14)	—	ND	ND	3.48 (0.72, 16.80)

NOTE: CI = confidence interval; ND = no data; and SMR = standardized mortality ratio.

[a]Leukemia 2- to 25-year follow-up, relative risk = 3.38 (90% CI 1.45–8.25).
[b]Data not presented.
[c]Malignant melanoma.

Darby and colleagues (1993a,b) studied mortality and cancer incidence in some 21,000 military participants (and 22,000 comparison subjects) in nuclear weapons tests conducted by the United Kingdom in Australia and the Pacific during the 1950s and 1960s. The study included data on deaths occurring through 1990, extending the follow-up period reported in their earlier study an additional 7 years (Darby et al., 1988a,b). Test participants had significantly increased leukemia mortality during the entire follow-up period (RR 1.75; CI 1.01–3.06), with a stronger effect observed for the period 2–25 years after exposure (RR 3.38; CI 1.45–8.25) than for the entire follow-up period. The investigators suggested that this elevation may be due to the low rates of leukemia seen in the comparison group during both follow-up periods, but did not rule out the possibility that exposure to radiation from nuclear tests may have had an effect on the leukemia risk, particularly during the earlier post-exposure period.

Pearce and colleagues (1996, 1997) investigated mortality and cancer incidence (through 1992) among 528 New Zealand participants (and 1,504 comparison subjects) in United Kingdom nuclear weapons tests conducted in the Pacific in 1957 and 1958. Leukemia (RR 5.59; CI 1.04–41.7) and the total hematologic cancer group (RR 3.75; CI 1.36–10.8) mortality rates were statistically significantly elevated. All-cause and all-cancer mortality were slightly elevated, but did not reach statistical significance.

Johnson and colleagues (1996) at the Medical Follow-up Agency of the Institute of Medicine investigated the mortality experience of more than 38,000 U.S. Navy personnel who participated in Operation Crossroads, a 1946 atmospheric nuclear test series that took place at the Bikini Atoll in the Pacific, and roughly 35,000 comparison personnel. The mortality experience of participants was evaluated relative to that of a comparison group, selected to be similar to the participants in several key ways—such as branch of service, time and location of service, age, and paygrade—but who had not participated in the Crossroads nuclear test series. Analysis found a slight but statistically significant increased risk of all-cause mortality among participants (RR 1.05; CI 1.02–1.07). Neither leukemia (RR 1.02; CI 0.75–1.39) nor all-cancer (RR 1.01; CI 0.96– 1.07) mortality were significantly elevated among Navy Crossroads participants.

In summary, the four studies of military personnel participating in atmospheric tests conducted by New Zealand, the United Kingdom, and the United States report rather consistent findings. For all-cause mortality, rate ratios from all four studies were slightly elevated (above 1.0). Two of those studies showed statistically significant estimated increased risk to participants. For all-cancer mortality, three studies reported elevated mortality rates and one study showed a decreased rate; none of these rates was statistically different from 1.0. Three studies reported elevated estimated risk of leukemia mortality among participants, relative to comparisons; two of these were statistically significant. Based largely on the findings from these studies of low-level radiation exposure in military populations, but also based on what is generally known about radiation effects, our study has focused on all-cause, all-cancer, and leukemia mortality as primary endpoints (see Chapter 9).

3

An Overview of the U.S. Nuclear Weapons Testing Program

From the start of the Trinity project in 1945 until the signing of the Limited Nuclear Test Ban Treaty in 1963, the United States conducted 19 operations (test series) involving tests of atmospheric nuclear weapons. In the course of these operations, more than 230 detonations (shots) were carried out, primarily at the Nevada Test Site and the Pacific Proving Ground (Gladeck and Johnson, 1996).[1] It is estimated that more than 200,000 Department of Defense (DoD) personnel, both military and civilian, participated in these tests (DTRA, 1999).

Responsibility for the planning and conduct of U.S. atmospheric nuclear weapons tests was shared by the DoD and the Atomic Energy Commission (AEC) (DNA, 1981), the successor to the Manhattan Engineer District (Gladeck and Johnson, 1996) and the predecessor of the Nuclear Regulatory Commission. The AEC was responsible for the development of nuclear technology, whereas the DoD was responsible for incorporating this technology into the United States military defense program (Harris et al., 1981). DoD military personnel (Army, Navy, Air Force, and Marine Corps members), as well as civilian employees and contractors of the DoD and AEC, all participated in nuclear weapons tests (DNA, 1981). The types of personnel present and the nature of their involvement in these tests varied by shot and by series.

In general, the roles and functions of DoD personnel present at test detonations were to witness the nuclear weapon test event, to participate in military exercises and perform tactical functions or support services, and to set up various scientific experiments and collect post-shot data. Dose limits in place during the tests functioned as safety guidelines rather than as restrictive cut-points.

---

[1] The Pacific Proving Ground tests took place on the Enewetak and Bikini Atolls, southwest of Hawaii.

These DoD-prescribed exposure limits varied, but generally allowed maximum exposures of 3 to 5 rem (30 to 50 millisievert [mSv]) "per test or series" (Gladeck and Johnson, 1996, p. 20). The Defense Nuclear Agency estimates that the average dose received by a participant was about 6 mSv (DTRA, 1999)— approximately twice as large as the average annual natural background dose received by a person living in the United States (NCRP, 1987) and more than 16 times lower than the threshold for deterministic effects (ICRP, 1984). It is estimated that less than 1 percent of all test participants received doses in excess of 50 mSv (DTRA, 1999), the current annual dose limit for radiation workers (CFR, 1991; Gladeck and Johnson, 1996).

Operations GREENHOUSE, UPSHOT-KNOTHOLE, CASTLE, REDWING, and PLUMBBOB represent a subset of the 19 total nuclear weapons test series. These five series included 62 shots and involved approximately 68,168 military participants (DSWA, 1997). The subset of five series was selected by the Medical Follow-up Agency's Subcommittee on Exposure at Tests of Nuclear Weapons as the focus of the 1985 National Research Council report *Mortality of Nuclear Weapons Test Participants* (Robinette et al., 1985). These particular series were chosen to include similar numbers of Nevada Test Site and Pacific Proving Ground participants. The availability and quality of both personnel and radiation dosimetry records were also considered in the selection of series for study (Robinette et al., 1985). Three of the five series were noted in the 1985 National Research Council report as including shots in which unexpected potential for radiation exposure arose during the test event (Robinette et al., 1985). PLUMBBOB, the series that includes Shot SMOKY, the exposure that was first identified as associated with leukemia, was also among the series selected for study. The present investigation is intended to supersede the 1985 study (see Chapter 1) and focuses, therefore, on the same subset of test series.

GREENHOUSE

Operation GREENHOUSE, the fourth postwar atmospheric nuclear weapons test series, was conducted in April and May of 1951 at the Pacific Proving Ground. GREENHOUSE consisted of four shots, all detonated on towers. Shots ranged in yield from 45.5 to 225 kilotons (kt) (Gladeck and Johnson, 1996).

Three of the four detonations resulted in significant downwind fallout that affected nearby ships and island base camps during the detonation and fallout periods (Berkhouse et al., 1983; Gladeck and Johnson, 1996). The DNA reports that fallout exposures were greater for island-based personnel than for shipboard personnel because water washdown systems, shielding, and decontamination procedures on board ships served to mitigate contamination (Berkhouse et al., 1983; DNA, 1981; Gladeck and Johnson, 1996). Approximately 9,528 personnel participated in this series (DSWA, 1997).[2] Navy personnel were present at

[2] Estimates presented in this overview reflect military personnel only.

GREENHOUSE shots in the largest number. Air Force and Army personnel were represented in smaller numbers, with few Marine Corps participants (DSWA, 1997).

UPSHOT-KNOTHOLE

Operation UPSHOT-KNOTHOLE was conducted between March and June of 1953 at the Nevada Test Site. During UPSHOT-KNOTHOLE, 11 nuclear devices were detonated—one device fired from a 280-millimeter cannon, three air drops, and seven tower shots. Shots in this series ranged in yield from 0.2 to 61 kt (Ponton et al., 1982). Nine of the tests in this series had yields in excess of 10 kt (Gladeck and Johnson, 1996).

During Shot BADGER, one of the tower detonations, wind shifts resulted in the exposure of members of the Marine Corps' First Battalion to higher than approved doses (DNA, 1982). Also, some of the military personnel present at shots in this series were exposed to neutron radiation while at positions relatively close to ground zero. Johnson and colleagues (1986) stated that "[d]uring Operations UPSHOT-KNOTHOLE (1953), TEAPOT (1955), and PLUMBBOB (1957), all at the Nevada Test Site, about 10,000 military observers and maneuvers troops were exposed to neutron radiation while observing tests from forward locations in the shot areas" (p. 21). Neutron doses for all but 544 participants were calculated to be less than 5 mSv (Gladeck and Johnson, 1996; Johnson et al., 1986). Altogether, approximately 18,473 personnel participated in shots in the UPSHOT-KNOTHOLE series (DSWA, 1997). Most participants were members of the Army, but small contingents of Marine Corps and Air Force personnel, and an even smaller number of Navy personnel, were also present (DSWA, 1997).

CASTLE

The CASTLE series was conducted to test large-yield thermonuclear devices. Operation CASTLE took place at the Pacific Proving Ground in March through May of 1954 and consisted of six test detonations, ranging in magnitude from 110 kt to 15 megatons (Mt). Shot BRAVO, the first detonation, significantly exceeded its expected yield and "was the largest device ever detonated by the U.S. Government as part of atmospheric nuclear weapons testing" (Gladeck and Johnson, 1996). Unexpectedly heavy fallout affected a small number of U.S. military personnel and the Japanese fishing boat *Fortunate Dragon No. 5* (Martin and Rowland, 1982). "Shot BRAVO was without question the worst single incident of fallout exposures in all the U.S. atmospheric testing program" (Martin and Rowland, 1982, p. 235). No other test in the series resulted in significant unexpected exposures (DNA, 1982; Martin and Rowland, 1982).

Most of the estimated 15,685 personnel (DSWA, 1997) participating in the CASTLE tests were members of the Navy. Sizable numbers of Air Force and

Army personnel were also present, as were a comparatively small number of Marines (DSWA, 1997).

REDWING

REDWING was a 17-detonation nuclear weapons test series conducted at the Pacific Proving Ground in the spring and summer of 1956. Like those in the CASTLE series, these detonations were conducted primarily as tests of thermonuclear devices (Bruce-Henderson et al., 1982). REDWING tests included six barge shots, three surface shots, six tower shots, and two air drops, ranging in magnitude from 13.7 kt to 5 Mt.

Because of the complications associated with Shot BRAVO in the CASTLE series, additional safety precautions were taken (Martin and Rowland, 1982), and dosimeters were issued to all participants in Operation REDWING (Bruce-Henderson et al., 1982). This operation "ran smoothly except for two incidents" (Bruce-Henderson et al., 1982, p. 3). One of the airdrops, Shot CHEROKEE, detonated considerably off target although no unexpected radiation exposures occurred as a result (Bruce-Henderson et al., 1982). Shot TEWA, fired at Bikini Atoll, resulted in fallout on the Enewetak base camp. Personnel remaining in the camp at the time of the test were unexpectedly exposed to ionizing radiation (Bruce-Henderson et al., 1982).

Approximately 12,923 personnel participated in the REDWING series (DSWA, 1997). Navy personnel constituted the largest group of armed forces personnel present during the test series. Army and Air Force, and to a lesser extent Marine Corps, personnel were also present (DSWA, 1997).

PLUMBBOB

Operation PLUMBBOB was conducted between May and October 1957 at the Nevada Test Site. PLUMBBOB consisted of 30 test events, including 24 nuclear detonations and 6 safety tests. Detonations ranged in yield from slight (safety tests) to 44 kt. Safety tests were designed to ensure the stability of the explosive components of nuclear devices prior to transport and stockpiling (Harris et al., 1981).

The opportunity for radiation exposure among participants in this test series was diffuse since "it was customary to offer personnel not assigned onsite duties (e.g., finance) the opportunity to watch a shot in the test series which they supported" (Harris et al., 1981). As with shots in the UPSHOT-KNOTHOLE series, some of the military observers and maneuvers personnel present at PLUMBBOB were exposed to neutron radiation while at positions relatively close to ground zero; however, radiation exposures of unexpected location or magnitude are not specifically noted for shots in this series. Concern regarding leukemia incidence among participants at Shot SMOKY in this series gave rise to studies of the health consequences of participation in atmospheric nuclear weapons tests.

Most of the estimated 11,559 (DSWA, 1997) PLUMBBOB participants were Army personnel. Members of the Marine Corps and Air Force participated in large numbers. A small number of Navy personnel were also involved in PLUMBBOB tests (DSWA, 1997).

ESTIMATES OF EXTERNAL DOSES

Although we did not use NTPR dose estimates in this study's analyses, we present in Table 3-1 (see page 18) the official published NTPR summary external dose data for each of the five series we studied for reference.

TABLE 3-1. Nuclear Test Personnel Review Program-Provided Summary of External Doses (in rem) for Atmospheric Nuclear Test Participants as of 30 September 1993, in Percentage of Series Participants

	Dose (rem)							
Series	0	>0–0.5	>0.5–1.0	>1.0–3.0	>3.0–5.0	>5.0–10.0	>10.0	Total
GREENHOUSE	15.8	15.8	11.4	33.5	21.0	2.2	0.1	99.8
UPSHOT-KNOTHOLE	4.2	29.9	8.8	38.7	17.5	0.7	0.0	99.8
CASTLE	5.3	40.7	17.7	27.3	6.0	2.8	0.3	100.1
REDWING	8.0	27.6	23.1	28.0	12.0	1.2	0.1	100.0
PLUMBBOB	22.3	52.4	16.5	7.7	0.7	0.3	0.0	99.9
Total	10.2	34.5	15.5	27.3	11.0	1.3	0.1	99.9

SOURCE: Gladeck and Johnson, 1996—*For the Record*, Table 1-4, p. 18.

4

Data Sources

The assembled information for this epidemiologic study comes from more than 100 distinct sources. Handwritten paper logs, microfilm or microfiche, computer files, medical records, work orders, transport orders, memoirs, interoffice memoranda, testimony, secondary compilations of primary sources, letters from spouses, death certificates, film badge records, computer programs, and benefits and compensation claims represent a diverse sample.

In this chapter, we describe the sources of data and their general limitations and assets. These data formed the basis of efforts to (1) identify individual members of the two study cohorts, (2) ensure the comparability of these cohorts, (3) ascertain vital status and mortality information, and (4) compare the mortality experience of those cohorts while controlling for characteristics of individuals, military service, or time period that might influence mortality.

Study staff, as well as DoD staff and contractors, made strenuous attempts to identify the existence of any relevant records, to acquire these records, and to corroborate information using multiple sources. Data related to personnel movements, radiation exposure, and vital status proved to be dispersed across the nation in cartons, computers, and file cabinets under the authority of many federal, state, and local agencies.

The following federal agencies and facilities maintain collections that the study staff used: the Department of Defense, including the Navy, Army, Air Force, and Marines, and the Nuclear Test Personnel Review Program of the Defense Threat Reduction Agency (DTRA);* the Department of Veterans Affairs

*The organizational locus of the Nuclear Test Personnel Review Program within the Department of Defense has been the Defense Nuclear Agency (until June 1996), the Defense Special Weapons Agency (until October 1998), and, currently, the Defense Threat Reduction Agency.

(VA), including its benefit and health components; the Department of Health and Human Services, including the National Center for Health Statistics, which maintains the National Death Index; and the National Archives and Records Administration's National Personnel Records Center, regional records centers, and the National Archives. Table 4-1 displays the relationships between the various sources and the data elements they yielded.

COHORT IDENTIFICATION

Nuclear Test Personnel Review Program

The source of information on participant identification and radiation exposure is the database maintained by DTRA—the NTPR database. The nature of this database and its implications for the design of the present study are described in this section.

In 1978, shortly after the Defense Nuclear Agency (now DTRA) became the executive agency for matters pertaining to the participation of DoD personnel in atmospheric nuclear tests, it officially established the NTPR program. The primary purposes of the NTPR were threefold: (1) to identify DoD personnel present at each test site and estimate their radiation exposures; (2) to identify the radiation monitoring measures that were in effect at the time of the tests; and (3) to develop a history of every atmospheric nuclear event that involved DoD personnel (Johnson et al., 1986). Initially, DNA directed the individual military services to conduct the NTPR research pertinent to their respective services, but in 1987 it consolidated the individual efforts into a single team effort.

The principal sources of information for the NTPR teams were the various military records available for review. Each branch of service has historical records, although not all in the same format. The Navy has deck logs that list officers and muster rolls that list enlisted personnel; Marine information comes from personnel rosters and daily diaries. Army and Air Force records are morning reports and personnel rosters. Personnel records from the National Personnel Records Center (NPRC) in St. Louis, Missouri, were also examined, where appropriate, to augment individual identifications. Not all Army and Air Force personnel records were available, however, because many were destroyed in a 1973 fire. Another source of information for the NTPR program has been a nationwide toll-free call-in program set up by DNA for veterans of atmospheric nuclear tests to report their participation (1-800-462-3683).

The NTPR-provided data tapes included name; military service number(s); date of birth; Social Security number(s); sex; paygrade, rank, or rating at series; unit membership during participation; permanent unit; and dates of entry into and separation from the service, among others. Names and service numbers are the primary concern of the NTPR program; the availability of the additional pieces of information is limited. For example, Social Security numbers are missing for the majority (55.6%) of personnel and dates of birth for approximately one-third.

National Archives and Military Collections

To select military units as potential sources of comparison cohort membership, JAYCOR, a DTRA contractor, reviewed Station Lists. Data on the individuals in the units chosen were obtained from military records such as deck logs and morning reports, as described earlier.

CHARACTERISTICS OF COHORT MEMBERS, INCLUDING DATE OF BIRTH AND VITAL STATUS

To permit vital status ascertainment of the military record-identified members of the participant and comparison cohorts, date of birth is essential and Social Security number is valuable. The main sources of these pieces of information are the VA Beneficiary Identification and Records Locator Subsystem (BIRLS), the VA Master Index (VAMI), and individual military personnel records.

Beneficiary Identification and Records Locator Subsystem

The sole source of mortality ascertainment in this study was the VA BIRLS database. It contains, among other things, identifying information on individuals who have submitted claims for veterans' benefits. BIRLS data were used in this study to verify information from military rosters, such as spelling of names, and to acquire date of birth, date of death, and the location of the claims record folder (from which the death certificate is retrieved). The key identifiers used in the BIRLS search are first and last names and military service number.

A veteran's death is noted in the VA records system if a claim is filed for death-related benefits, such as reimbursement for burial expense or burial in a national cemetery. Eligibility is determined by various factors including time of service, service-connected disability, cause of death, and financial resources of the veteran's estate. The eligibility rules were modified by legislation in 1981, making benefits more restrictive than earlier, which may have affected the number and characteristics of veterans whose deaths are reported to VA and recorded in BIRLS. When a death benefit is claimed for a veteran, the VA requires a copy of the death certificate for claim processing. The death certificate then becomes part of the veteran's claims folder, which eventually is retired to the federal archives records centers.

TABLE 4-1. Sources of Data Items

Source of Data	Name	Military Service Number	Social Security Number	Series Participation	Part. Unit	Perm. Unit	Rank, Rating, or Paygrade	Dates of Service	Dose	Claims Folder Location or ID	Date of Birth	Fact of Death	Date of Death	Cause of Death
DoD														
NTPR[a]		+	+	+	+	+	+	+	+		+			
Navy Yard[b]	+	+			+		+							
VA														
BIRLS[c]		+	+							+	+	+	+	
VAMI[d]	+	+								+			+	
VBA													+	+
VARos[e]														
NARA[f]														
Archives[g]	+	+			+		+							
FARCs[h]											+		+	+
NPRC[i]														
Assorted[j]	+	+			+		+			+				
Personnel record[k]											+			
DHHS														
NDI[l]											+	x	+	x

NOTE: Part. Unit = participating unit; Perm. Unit = permanent unit; "+" indicates a data source used for analysis; and "x" indicates a data source used only in validation exercises. DHHS = Department of Health and Human Services; DoD = Department of Defense; NARA = National Archives and Records Administration; and VA = Department of Veterans Affairs.

[a] Nuclear Test Personnel Review Program, Defense Threat Reduction Agency, DoD (DTRA used 99 data sources).
[b] Navy Yard (muster rolls, rosters, etc., for some Marine units).
[c] Beneficiary Identification and Records Locator Subsystem, VA (since 1972; automated and targeted access).
[d] VA Master Index (1917 to January 1972; index cards on microfilm).
[e] Veterans Benefits Administration regional offices, VA (active VA claims folders).
[f] National Archives and Records Administration.
[g] National Archives at College Park, NARA (deck logs, muster rolls, etc., for Navy units).
[h] Federal archives and records centers, NARA (retired VA claims folders, which remain under VA jurisdiction).
[i] National Personnel Records Center, St. Louis, Mo.
[j] Assorted archived records (personnel rosters and morning reports for Army and Air Force units; and some Marine unit diaries).
[k] Military personnel records (transferred from branch of service to NPRC).
[l] National Death Index, National Center for Health Statistics, DHHS (deaths 1979 and later).

VA Master Index

The VA Master Index (VAMI) was the predecessor of BIRLS. From 1917 to January 1972, VA created an index card for each veteran who applied for any benefit, including insurance, education and home loans, health care, and disability compensation. These VAMI cards have since been transferred to microfilm. Because the BIRLS database was not created directly from VAMI, some references to pre-1972 deaths can be found in VAMI but not BIRLS. Therefore, when no record for an individual could be found in the computerized BIRLS database, the microfilm copy of VAMI was searched. VAMI was also the source of additional identifying information such as an alias or a military service number that allowed a more accurate repeated search in BIRLS.

Military Personnel Folder

The military maintains a personnel record folder for each service member. The folders for those who served in the 1950s are archived at the National Personnel Records Center in St. Louis, Missouri. These records contain personal identification data, such as date of birth, military service numbers, and sometimes Social Security numbers, in a standardized format.

As mentioned previously, the availability of personnel records is limited; the fire at the NPRC in 1973 destroyed about 80 percent of the records for Army personnel discharged between November 1, 1912, and January 1, 1960, and about 75 percent of the records for Air Force personnel with surnames from “Hubbard” through “Z” discharged between September 25, 1947, and January 1, 1964. For most individuals whose personnel records were destroyed, their medical records, which were filed in the same folder, were also lost.

Social Security numbers were not routinely used in the military records system during 1951–1957; hence, a large yield was not expected from these sources. Because of concerns regarding completeness of death reporting by BIRLS and differential characteristics between the deaths found and not found by BIRLS (Boyle and Decoufle, 1990; Page, 1992), the National Death Index, maintained by the National Center on Health Statistics, a non-VA source, was searched to validate BIRLS-based vital status ascertainment (see Chapter 9 for details).

CAUSE OF DEATH

Veteran's Claim Folder

Once a veteran's death had been identified through a BIRLS search, a copy of the death certificate was requested from the VA regional office (VARO) or the regional federal archives records center (FARC) noted as the claims folder location in BIRLS. Obtaining death certificate copies from these sources is a time-consuming process. MFUA staff has estimated that about 70 percent of the death certificates are obtained within six months after the initial request is submitted. For the remaining 30 percent, however, the process may take years.

National Death Index

When, after reasonable effort, a death certificate could not be obtained from the VARO or FARC, information on the individual was submitted to the National Death Index (NDI) with a request for cause-of-death information. NDI is a computer database maintained at the National Center for Health Statistics. Compiled from data tapes submitted by each state's vital statistics office, it contains identifying information on all U.S. deaths since 1979. Researchers can get the state and death certificate number of a known death and then request the death certificate from the state. Since 1998, through the NDI-Plus program, researchers can request the death certificate information directly from NDI. The NDI-Plus computer tape includes name, date of birth, date of death, and underlying and associated causes of death, as recorded on the death certificate.

Although we used NDI cause of death in the study's analysis, we relied on its *fact-of-death* ascertainment only as a validation tool (see Chapter 8).

POPULATION MORTALITY RATES FOR COMPARISON

For the calculation of standardized mortality ratios for each cohort, the University of Pittsburgh's Mortality Data and Population Statistics program created cause-specific mortality rates for the ages and calendar time of interest for each of the study cohorts, participant and referent. Although race and sex information was not available to us for the study cohort, we determined that *of the cohort deaths* less than half a percent were female and between 8 and 9 percent were black. With that data, along with historical anecdotal information about the military and the nuclear weapons program in the 1950s, we decided to use white male rates as an approximation to calculate expected mortality rates.

5

The Participant Cohort

The core of this report is a comparison of the mortality experience of nuclear test participants and a comparable referent group of nonparticipants. This section contains a description of the participant cohort selection process.

The participant cohort includes all military personnel identified by February 28, 1997, by the Defense Threat Reduction Agency (DTRA) as participants in at least one of the selected five series of U.S. atmospheric nuclear weapons tests. This study includes active duty personnel but does not include Reserve, National Guard, and Coast Guard personnel. The five test series—Operations GREENHOUSE, UPSHOT-KNOTHOLE, CASTLE, REDWING, and PLUMBBOB—are the same series that were examined in the 1985 Medical Follow-up Agency (MFUA) study.[1] As described earlier, these five series (consisting of 62 tests) were originally chosen for study from the 19 U.S. atmospheric nuclear weapons test series. Their selection was based on the availability and quality of records for personnel identification and radiation dosimetry and a design based on comparable numbers of participants at tests conducted in the Pacific and the continental United States.

DTRA used the congressionally mandated and Department of Veterans Affairs-issued regulatory definition of *participant*: (1) any U.S. military personnel who were present at the test site or who performed official military duties in connection with ships, aircraft, or other equipment in direct support of an atmospheric nuclear test during its official operational period; (2) any U.S. military personnel who were present at the test site or other test staging area to perform official military duties in connection with completion of projects related to the nuclear test, including decontamination of equipment used for the test, dur

[1] See Chapter 1 for a discussion of the 1985 publication and the rationale for the new study.

ing the 6 months following the official period of an atmospheric nuclear test; or (3) any U.S. military personnel who served as members of the garrison or maintenance forces on Enewetak at any time from June 21, 1951, through July 1, 1952, after Operation GREENHOUSE; or from August 7, 1956, through August 7, 1957, after Operation REDWING (CFR, 1998a). Personnel in the last group, although not fitting the standard definition of test participation, were included by Congress and VA regulation as if they were participants because GREENHOUSE Shot ITEM and REDWING Shot TEWA, fired at Bikini Atoll, resulted in fallout on the Enewetak base camp, causing radiation exposure among DoD personnel who remained in the camp (Gladeck and Johnson, 1996; JAYCOR, 1995).

Table 5-1 displays the operational period and the 6-month post-operational period for each of the five series.

Identifying test participants was a difficult task, however, because a complete roster of test participants did not exist and the permanent DoD records of atmospheric tests did not contain the necessary identification information. Therefore, NTPR conducted large-scale searches of historical records, ranging from federal archives and records centers to private collections (Gladeck and Johnson, 1996). For example, the Navy NTPR procedure for identifying participants was first to identify the participating ships and squadrons through available historical records. Deck logs, along with muster rolls and daily diaries, were then located to identify individual participants. For Army and Air Force NTPR teams, morning reports and personnel rosters of the units were located.

Another source of information for the NTPR program has been a nationwide toll-free call-in program set up by DNA for veterans of the atmospheric nuclear tests to report details of their participation in any test. When a call is received from a veteran or veteran's representative, an NTPR interviewer asks a standard set of questions and files the information. If a review of available records confirms the veteran's participation in the nuclear test series, the verified information is added to a computerized file that contains the participant data obtained primarily through record reviews. It is the latter, record-based file, rather than the initial direct contact, that is the source of data on participant identification for the current study.

When the 1985 study began, individual NTPR teams were still rapidly identifying test participants. Since 1987, when DNA consolidated the service NTPR teams into a single operation, identification of new participants has slowed, but continues; participating units continue to be identified using newly discovered historical records, and the inclusion criteria for classifying participants have been broadened.

TABLE 5-1. Official Operational and Postoperational Periods for the Five Series

		End Date		
Operation	Start Date	Official Operation	Postoperational Period	Garrison or Maintenance Forces on Enewetak
GREENHOUSE	April 8, 1951	June 20, 1951	December 21, 1951	July 1, 1952
UPSHOT-KNOTHOLE	March 17, 1953	June 20, 1953	December 21, 1953	NA
CASTLE	March 1, 1954	May 31, 1954	November 30, 1954	NA
REDWING	May 5, 1956	August 6, 1956	February 7, 1957	August 7, 1957
PLUMBBOB	May 28, 1957	October 22, 1957	April 23, 1958	NA

NOTE: NA = not applicable.

SOURCE: CFR, 1998b, and JAYCOR, 1995.

TABLE 5-2. Estimates and Determined Extent of Participant Misclassification in the 1985 Dataset

Assessed Misclassification	GAO[a]	OTA[b]	1999 Report[c]
1985 Report Total	46,186	46,186	49,148[d]
Wrongly included	14,854	4,500	8,877
Wrongly omitted	28,215	15,000	24,161
"Correct" total	59,547	56,686	64,432
Additions due to decision change, not error			3,736
Total			68,168

[a] General Accounting Office (1992).
[b] U.S. Congress Office of Technology Assessment (Gelband, 1992).
[c] Medical Follow-up Agency use of rosters supplied by the Nuclear Test Personnel Review Program as of 1997.
[d] The data file for 1985 included 49,148 records, 2,962 of which were excluded due to problem data.

From December 1993 through March 1997, DTRA transmitted to MFUA progressively updated data tapes that identified participants in the five series. Because MFUA was revisiting the questions first considered in the 1985 study, primarily because of inaccuracies in the DTRA-provided participant roster used in the 1985 analysis, both MFUA and DTRA provided intense and ongoing scrutiny of roster identification for the current study.[2]

RELATIONSHIP OF PARTICIPANT ROSTERS USED IN THE 1985 PUBLICATION AND THIS REPORT

In the early 1990s, DTRA (then the Defense Nuclear Agency) announced that the personnel dataset it had provided MFUA contained substantial errors of inclusion and exclusion. Because this dataset was the basis of MFUA's Five Series Study published in 1985, the U.S. General Accounting Office, the congressional Office of Technology Assessment, members of the U.S. Senate and House of Representatives, and MFUA itself recommended redoing the mortality analyses using a corrected dataset. MFUA further enhanced the study design (partially in response to criticism of the 1985 report) to include a military comparison cohort.

Table 5-2 displays the extent of overlap between the participant cohort used for the 1985 publication and the cohort on which this current study is based. Eighty-four percent of the 1985 cohort is included in the current list. However, these people comprise only 57 percent of the current list. If we were to exclude

[2] Appendix D reviews the work done to validate participant cohort membership.

from this calculation the 3,736 personnel included in the current list solely because of their presence in post-series rosters—reflecting a post-1985 change in inclusion criteria rather than identification errors—we still see that 60 percent of the current cohort was in the 1985 cohort.

PARTICIPATION IN SERIES OTHER THAN THE SELECTION SERIES

Participants were chosen for this study if they were assigned to military units that participated in at least one of the five selected series. The *selection series* is the first, chronologically, of the five series to which a member of the participant cohort could have been assigned. Three percent of this cohort participated in more than one of the five series and some participated in series other than the five. Table 5-3 illustrates, for the participant cohort, by selection series, the distribution of other test participation, according to the NTPR database. The count includes the five series studied in this report, any of the other 14 test series, and assignment to Hiroshima or Nagasaki.[3]

[3] Although Hiroshima and Nagasaki were not test series, individuals who were assigned to units in these areas in time proximate to the atomic bomb detonations are included in the NTPR database.

TABLE 5-3. Total Number of Series in Which Members of Each Selection Series Participated

	Selection Series					All Participants	
No. of Participation Series	GREENHOUSE	UPSHOT-KNOTHOLE	CASTLE	REDWING	PLUMBBOB	No.	%
Selection series only	7,289	16,840	13,076	10,536	10,735	58,476	85.8
+ 1 other series	1,778	1,255	2,158	2,048	675	7,914	11.6
+ 2 other series	302	233	362	223	125	1,245	1.8
+ 3 other series	87	79	62	77	18	323	0.5
+ 4 other series	35	32	18	33	4	122	0.2
+ 5 other series	15	18	2	6	1	42	0.1
+ 6 other series	11	8	7		1	27	0.0
+ 7 other series	3	5				8	0.0
+ 8 other series	4	1				5	0.0
+ 9 other series	3	2				5	0.0
+ 10 other series						0	—
+ 11 other series						0	—
+ 12 other series	1					1	0.0
Total	9,528	18,473	15,685	12,923	11,559	68,168	100.0

6

The Referent Cohort

To determine whether participants at the five nuclear test series had different mortality experience than a comparable group of nonparticipants, we built a comparison referent cohort of nonparticipants. Using records kept by the Department of Defense and the National Archives and Records Administration, we used frequency matching to assemble a referent cohort that would be similar to the Defense Threat Reduction Agency (DTRA)-provided five-series participant cohort according to branch of service, time period, location (Pacific, western United States, other), age, type of unit, and paygrade. We did this by creating a pool of units—such as ships and battalions—from among those selected by DTRA as likely to be comparable. DTRA selected reference units by considering their similarity to the participating units. The similarity was defined by function, size, paygrade distribution, and time period. Units assigned to states downwind of the Nevada Test Site, to operations in Korea, or to participation in any atmospheric nuclear test were not eligible for selection.

From the eligible units, we selected individuals to fit the paygrade distribution of the participants in the related unit. Those participants without reasonably close referents in terms of paygrade were pooled by type of unit, within branch of service and series, as were the excess individuals in referent cohort units who were not selected. Individuals in each service were selected from the larger referent cohort pools to be similar in paygrade and unit type to the individuals remaining in the participant pool.

MFUA, with DTRA assistance, assembled a 64,781-member military reference cohort. Reference individuals were selected using frequency matching on the following criteria: (1) service during the 12 months immediately preceding or following the date of the participant's selection series, (2) service in a similar unit in the same branch of service as the participant during the test period, (3) the same or similar paygrade at the time as the participant during the test period, and (4) no participation in any atmospheric nuclear weapons testing program.

Since no single source document can provide all of the information necessary for assembling the referent cohort, the assembly procedure was divided into three phases. The first phase involved selecting reference units; the second phase involved building a referent pool by identifying names, service numbers, and paygrades of all individuals in the units; and the third phase involved selecting individual referents and further obtaining identifying information concerning those individuals.

The NTPR team identified referent units through a review of Station Lists, which specify all units according to their numerical designation in each calendar year; these unit specifications can be cross-referenced with the unit's physical location.

The similarity between the participant and referent units was determined by considering their function, size, and paygrade distribution. Since unit names are usually consistent and can provide a basic understanding of these characteristics within the unit, the reference unit selection was based on unit names. The geographic area of the station was also considered in selecting reference units. Units stationed in Utah, Arizona, New Mexico, Colorado, and Nevada within 2 years of any atmospheric continental test were excluded from referent unit selection since they may have been exposed to test fallout. Units stationed in Korea during the Korean War (1950–1953) were also excluded. Units participating in any atmospheric nuclear weapon tests within a defined time period were excluded as well: for the Army and Marine Corps, units within a 2-year window of any test period; for the Air Force, units within a 3-year window; and for the Navy, units within a 4-year window. These time frames were chosen based on typical unit rotation periods within the services.

More than one reference unit was selected for each participating unit: two units for each participating unit in the Navy and Marine Corps; six units for each participating unit in the Army and Air Force. The principal purpose of obtaining multiple reference units was to provide a referent population pool large enough for frequency sampling on branch, series, and paygrade. These multiple units were ordered and sampled according first to geography and then to time, as indicated below. For continental tests, units stationed within the continental United States had a higher priority than those stationed outside the continental United States. For Pacific test series, similar units stationed within the Pacific theater had a higher priority than those outside the Pacific theater. Units stationed within the 6-month window of the test series period had a higher priority than those within the 12-month window. Therefore, for the continental tests, for example, units stationed in the continental United States within the 6-month window had the highest priority, followed by those stationed in the continental United States within the 12-month window.

The degree of difficulty in identifying reference units ranged from minimal to extreme. Finding reference units such as ships, battalions, and standard squadrons was relatively simple. However, finding counterparts of temporary units such as provisional, special project, and observer units, was difficult. The structure of these temporary units did not follow the established standards (e.g., tables of distribution and allowances, tables of organization and equipment); therefore, the unit names do not provide a basic description of their size, function, and paygrade distribution.

Once the reference units had been chosen, organizational records of each branch of service were reviewed to identify the names, service numbers, and paygrades of all personnel in these units. For the Navy, all enlisted men aboard a particular ship can be found in the ship's muster rolls (on microfilm); officers are listed in the ship's deck logs (in log books) and on post-1955 muster rolls; both sources are available through the National Archives. For Navy shore units, which do not have muster rolls and deck logs, unit diaries were reviewed to ascertain the identifiers of the unit members. For the Marine Corps, muster rolls (on microfilm) and Station Lists were searched to accurately identify military service numbers or names.

For the Army, monthly personnel rosters and morning reports that are available in the National Personnel Records Center (NPRC) in St. Louis were used. The morning reports have been completed each day since World War II, usually at the company level. They list persons who experienced a change in duty status, showing their names, service numbers, and ranks. A change in status could be discharge, temporary duty, absence, return from absence, reassignment, promotion, etc. Since the morning reports may list the same person multiple times and omit certain persons depending on their changes in duty status, the monthly personnel roster was used as the primary information source. For the Air Force, morning reports are the only available source.

Once the referent pool was constructed for each service, the roster was matched to the NTPR database on name and service number(s), to exclude those who are known to be participants in any atmospheric nuclear weapons test.

The members of the referent pool were grouped by unit and paygrade, as were members of the participating units. For each paygrade, the same number of reference subjects as participants was selected according to the unit priority order described earlier. When there were insufficient numbers of referent pool members in a specific paygrade, an adjacent paygrade was used.

Table 6-1 shows the closeness of matching. Selection categories 1 and 2—in which service, series, paygrade, and type of unit are all exact matches—account for 79.5 percent of the study population. Another 15.5 percent was selected using one of six close, although not exact, combinations of characteristics outlined in the table. The pool of potential referent personnel did not include, however, sufficient numbers of certain participant characteristic combinations for there to be equal numbers in each cohort. Each combination, however, is represented in both cohorts. The referent cohort has 3,388 fewer members than the participant cohort.

The referent cohort acquisition process yielded a group of individuals with distributions similar to the participant cohort for the desired and available characteristics. This balance within the overall and series-specific cohorts is illustrated in Chapter 10.

TABLE 6-1. Closeness of Frequency Matching in the Selection of Referent Cohort Members

Closeness of Frequency Matching Categories						
Order	No.	%	Service	Series	Paygrade	Unit
1 (best)	28,044	43.3	Exact*	Exact*	Exact*	Exact*
2	26,144	40.4	Exact	Exact	Exact	Same type of unit (types defined separately for each service)
3	4,129	6.4	Exact	Exact	Exact	Substituted (and grouped) type of unit
4	1,765	2.7	Exact	Exact	Defined paygrade groups (E1–E3, E4–E5, E6+, O1–O3, O4+, W1–W4)	Exact
5	3,956	6.1	Exact	Exact	Exact	None
6	207	0.3	Exact	UPSHOT-KNOTHOLE referents used for PLUMBBOB participants	Exact	Same type of unit (category)
7	396	0.6	Exact	UPSHOT-KNOTHOLE referents used for PLUMBBOB participants	Close paygrade groups (UK O3 referents used for PLUMBBOB O4–O5 participants)	Same type of unit (category)
8	140	0.2	Exact	Exact	Close paygrade groups (PLUMBBOB O3 referents used for PLUMBBOB O4–O5 participants)	Same type of unit (category)
Total	64,781	100.0				

*An exact match for "service" is selecting Air Force referents for Air Force participants; the same is true for "series" and "paygrade." For "unit," the specific unit has been selected that the Defense Threat Reduction Agency contractor recommended as matching the participant unit.

7

Exposure Definition and Measurement

The National Research Council's 1985 study (Robinette et al., 1985) of participants in the five nuclear weapons test series on which the current report focuses used dose data provided by the Defense Nuclear Agency's (DNA) Nuclear Test Personnel Review Program (NTPR). Using data painstakingly collected from diverse sources, NTPR staff and contractors attempted to assign to each individual participant a valid estimate of the radiation dose received (Gladeck and Johnson, 1996). Initial plans for the new Five Series Study included the use of these individual dose assignments.

The committee charged with oversight of the present study created a working group,* with external expertise, to review DNA dosimetry estimation procedures and results. Based on the working group's findings, the full committee issued a letter report (IOM, 1995; reprinted as Appendix A in this report), stating that the dosimetry estimates were not appropriate for dose–response analyses in the context of epidemiologic studies. In this chapter, we describe (1) the background and limits of the NTPR dosimetry work as it relates to this study's protocol, (2) alternative exposure surrogates considered, (3) decisions made for the analyses in this report, and (4) possibilities for further investigations.

---

*John Till, Ph.D., served as chair of the dosimetry working group, which included one other oversight committee member (Clarice Weinberg, Ph.D.) and three external dosimetry experts (F. Owen Hoffman, Ph.D.; Keith J. Schiager, Ph.D.; and John Taschner).

DNA-PROVIDED DOSE ESTIMATES

Individual Doses

The Nuclear Test Personnel Review (NTPR) database contains a dose assignment for each participant, derived in most cases through reconstruction based on duty assignments. In less than half of cases, the assigned dose is based on one or more film badges worn by the participant or on a film badge worn by another participant in the same unit (cohort badging).

Ideally, exposure measurements would be (1) individual-specific; (2) recorded by time, duration, and dose; (3) sensitive to different components of exposure (e.g., alpha, beta, or gamma radiation); (4) previously validated for use in similar situations; (5) quantitative and at least theoretically reproducible; (6) complete, in that they cover all exposures for all involved people; and (7) accepted by all interested parties. As stated above, based on our examination of the NTPR dosimetry data, we do not believe that these data are appropriate for the individual-specific assignments necessary for the type of epidemiologic comparisons on which this report is based.

A working group of the Five Series Study oversight committee assessed the basis and quality of the data upon which dose assignments were made and concluded that they were not suitable for dose–response analyses in epidemiology (IOM, 1995, p. 2):

> The Working Group concluded that there has been a lack of consistency over time in NTPR dose estimation methods and, in particular, in the methods of assigning "high-sided" doses, that is, doses in which uncertainties are resolved in favor of assigning higher doses rather than lower doses. In some cases, because of the existing compensation program, procedures for assigning doses have been different for those who did and did not file a claim for a radiogenic cancer. Neither the dose assignment methods nor the database itself are thoroughly documented. In addition, uncertainties have not been estimated in a consistent manner and do not incorporate all potential sources of variability inherent in the dosimetry.

The conclusions also state, "Although there is anecdotal evidence that individual doses may have been greatly underestimated in individual cases, the overall tendency may have been to overestimate both external and internal doses" (p. 13).

Individualized dose reconstructions are "generally only carried out if there is a specific institutional or legal need for a refined estimate" (p. 11)—for example, when a veteran or a survivor files a claim for health or death benefits. Because reconstructed doses are more likely to be overestimated than others (IOM, 1995), these NTPR doses differ systematically based on health status, which is closely tied to our study endpoints. We think that using them would introduce sufficient bias to render the epidemiologic analysis of these data useless. Veterans, mean while, have expressed concerns that the assigned doses are significantly lower than justified, based on their firsthand experiences at the test site.

Alternative Uses of Dose Data

We looked for other, indirect, quantitative dose measures obtainable from the NTPR database. We hypothesized that either the number of badges issued to an individual or the total dose derived from badge data might be a more reliable measure of individual exposure than the reconstructed total dose discussed above.

Based on DNA background material, we hypothesized that the participants most likely to be exposed to ionizing radiation would have been issued more badges than those believed less likely to be exposed. Facing the same dosimetry question in our earlier study of Operation CROSSROADS participation (Johnson et al., 1996), we had looked for relationships between the number of badges issued to an individual and both the total dose assigned to that individual and the dose assigned to the individual using badge data alone. Finding no relationship, we rejected using the number of badges as an exposure surrogate for the CROSSROADS study and, now, for this study as well.

The assignment of individual-level dose surrogates based on badged dose was also considered and rejected. The issuance of personal dosimeters varied by service and series. An estimated 45 percent of all atmospheric nuclear weapons test participants (DTRA, 1999), and 52 percent of all participants in the five test series in particular (IOM, 1995), have individual radiation dose information on record (see Appendix A). The REDWING series had the largest number of participants who were issued a personal dosimeter (82 percent), and UPSHOT-KNOTHOLE had the lowest (13 percent). This reflects a change in procedures over time, not a difference in the anticipated exposures. The value of the dosimetry information for use in epidemiologic studies is questionable, however, even in instances in which relatively high proportions of personnel were badged (IOM, 1995). Individuals who were badged did not wear their badges continuously during their exposure, according to participant and DTRA accounts. Thus, an individual's cumulative dose from film badges may well give an incomplete picture of total dose. We examined the CROSSROADS dosimetry data to determine if an individual's assigned dose and badged dose were proportional, which would allow an assumption that badges were indicative of the total dose accrued by the individual. We found that individuals with very similar badged totals had widely disparate assigned doses due to differing dose reconstructions.

Other approaches were considered and rejected. For example, we might use the highest recorded doses and the zero doses, hoping that dosimetry was more reliable at the extremes. However, the committee was concerned that the NTPR database did not adequately distinguish between truly zero doses and unknown or unmeasured doses.

Finally, we explored how one might use dosimetry as an *indicator* rather than a *measure* of radiation. Again, each approach to the development of an in dex of probable exposure that could be supported by the available dosimetry presented difficulties. In summary, seeing no evidence that the film badge data provided an exposure surrogate adequate for use in this study, we chose not to use them.

POTENTIAL SURROGATE MEASURES OF DOSE

After ruling out the use of DTRA-assigned doses, we considered various ways in which to categorize exposure. Some suggestions—such as number of series, number of individual shots, and type and size of detonation—were rejected immediately because this information did not correlate closely with what we know about dose. For example, an individual who was assigned to units at four different test series, but was assigned to indoor locations far from the detonations, might have received no radiation dose, whereas another individual who attended only one test shot may have had responsibilities within meters of ground zero soon after the detonation.

The number of series in which an individual participated and the individual's branch of service were rejected as dose surrogates for similar reasons. We did conduct some analyses in an attempt to determine whether certain series could be considered as proxies for exposure. The results of some of these analyses are presented in Appendix E. They provide descriptive information, but we believe that they are difficult to interpret because of the many unmeasured and potentially heterogeneous circumstances that they represent.

Given the wealth of anecdotal and written record descriptions of potential high-dose situations (e.g., troops involved in maneuvers such as Desert Rock Troop Brigades; those involved in cloud sampling; and radiation safety personnel), we discussed how we might use historical, qualitative information to define high-dose groups. Because these task groups often were not defined by a specific unit name, however, we could not identify which individuals to assign to the study category. Historical narrative records suggest that particular ships were subject to higher exposures than others; for example, individuals assigned to the USS *Bairoko*, USS *Philip*, Rongerik, Rongelap, or the boat pool. We could not look at RADSAFE (radiation safety) personnel for reasons of feasibility and interpretability. RADSAFE is not always a unit designation; radiation safety personnel may be spread out among other units and their potential exposures diluted by the lower doses of others in these units. Also, professional radiation experts may have used more safeguards (e.g., protection equipment) and received lower doses in exposure situations because of their expertise.

One distinction among the participants that may be exposure related is the location of the test series. The weapons tested in the Pacific and Nevada test areas were primarily two different types of devices. For the Pacific test areas, fusion weapons were tested primarily, and for the Nevada Test Site, fission devices. Although these types of weapons are fundamentally different in the interactions that led to detonation, the residual radiation fields created in the two locations are very similar. Nevertheless, because of environmental differences between the test areas and the tasks that personnel were expected to carry out, it is possible that the pathways of exposure were somewhat different. For example, military personnel who were exposed to radiation from contaminated ships in the Pacific tests were likely not to have received as much exposure via the inhalation pathway as their counterparts at the Nevada Test Site where resuspended particulate matter could have been inhaled. Another example of potential differences between exposures is the type of activities that servicemen were undertaking. In the Nevada tests, most personnel were exposed as a result of ground contamination in areas where they either witnessed the explosions or entered following the blasts. In the Pacific, many personnel were exposed after they went aboard ships that had been placed at varying distances from ground zero. Although it would be expected that the predominant exposure at both test areas would have been direct gamma radiation originating from surfaces, differences likely existed in the radiation dose fields and thus could have exposed some organs of the body in different ways.

Although these scenarios of exposure between the two test areas are speculation, it is evident that the two environments within which servicemen were working differed greatly and these differences could have led to exposure being created and received in different ways. These potential differences in exposure suggest that there may be justification for considering a comparison between disease among veterans who received the majority of their dose from one location or the other. The Five Series Study design purposefully included participants from both land and sea test sites.

DECISIONS FOR THE ANALYSES IN THIS REPORT

Based on the considerations described in the preceding sections, the committee and staff decided not to use dosimetry data in the analysis. This decision was not taken lightly. The painstaking effort to develop the dose data was immense. The dose data, however, as previously described, do contain systematic differences that could affect the study's results in ways that are not well defined. Therefore, without looking at dose–outcome correlations, we made the decision not to use the individual-specific reconstructed or badged doses.

The core study, therefore, is a comparison of the participant and referent cohorts. Status as a participant is taken to be the most reliable (though broad) indicator of exposure. The participant versus referent cohort dichotomy provides the largest group of people to study, size being important when considering rare outcomes such as leukemia. Using participant status to represent exposure—in this case, potential exposure to ionizing radiation and possibly to other test-related environmental factors—also presents many limitations regarding epidemiologic study. We cannot account for differences in potential radiation exposure among participants or their exposure to other ill-defined environmental or occupational factors, either related to or independent of nuclear test participation (e.g., later employment as a radiological technician or a radiation worker in the nuclear power industry).

FUTURE OPTIONS FOR USE OF DOSIMETRY

Should the current study yield interesting findings, the oversight committee has discussed further avenues of research. Demonstrating an association between dose and outcome would greatly support any finding of higher mortality among participants than referents. Once a specific outcome is selected (which was not feasible in this study because of the requirement that all participants and a range of outcomes be considered), an efficient design such as the nested case-control study could be used. Such studies require fewer subjects, making less prohibitive, for example, the per-person expense of custom dose reconstruction. For reasons explained in detail in its earlier report (IOM, 1995), the oversight committee believes that useful dose reconstructions can be achieved if certain guidelines—such as unbiased selection of participants and technical consistency in methodology for dose estimation—are followed.

8

Mortality Ascertainment

Do atomic test participants have a reduced life expectancy compared to non-participants? Are they at increased risk for certain causes of death? Could this be related to radiation exposure? Our basis for addressing these questions is a comparison of death rate, timing, and cause of death for the two cohorts. Correct ascertainment of mortality data, therefore, is crucial to the validity of this epidemiologic study. In this chapter, we first describe ascertainment methods, verification activities, and validation analyses, and then proceed to an assessment of success.

FACT-OF-DEATH ASCERTAINMENT

As described in Chapter 4, the Department of Veterans Affairs (VA) Beneficiary Identification and Records Locator Subsystem (BIRLS) is the sole source of fact-of-death ascertainment for this report's dataset. If a person's record was not found in the BIRLS database, the VA Master Index was searched for additional descriptive information (e.g., military service number or a middle name) that might allow a connection to a BIRLS record. BIRLS information, then, results in a defined set of possible mortality ascertainment outcomes:

- known dead—indication of death in the BIRLS database, and
- not known dead—no indication of death in the BIRLS database.

Each of these is composed of subgroups described by the availability of other pieces of information. An individual is classified as *known dead* if the BIRLS database (1) explicitly refers to a death, giving a date or a cause, or (2) lists the location of the VA claims folder as the federal archives. *Not known dead* is the accurate way of referring to individuals who in other studies might be classified as "alive" or "lost to follow-up." What we do know about these individuals is that either the BIRLS database (1) has a record of the individual but no reference to death or federal archives or (2) contains no reference at all to the individual.

The BIRLS procedure identified 38,055 deaths among the 132,949 members of the two cohorts. The 1,865 of these deaths that occurred after our defined end of follow-up (December 31, 1996) were treated as alive for the analyses presented in this report. Establishing a calendar cutoff of dates of death is necessary to allow time for adequate cause-of-death follow-up activities. The remaining 36,190 deaths constitute 27.2 percent of the combined cohorts.

Table 8-1 and Table 8-2 present the vital status categories for the participant and referent cohorts.

TABLE 8-1. Vital Status as of December 31, 1996

	Participants (n = 68,168)		Referents (n = 64,781)		Total (n = 132,949)	
Vital Status	No.	% of Cohort	No.	% of Cohort	No.	% of Cohort
Not known dead (no)	49,651	72.8	47,108	72.7	96,759	72.8
Known to be dead (yes)	18,517	27.2	17,673	27.3	36,190	27.2
Total	68,168	100.0	64,781	100.0	132,949	100.0

FACT-OF-DEATH VALIDATION

BIRLS is the only source of fact of death in this study. How complete is BIRLS as a record of veterans' deaths? If it does not capture almost all deaths, mortality studies based on these data would be inaccurate. If it captures certain kinds of deaths or deaths of certain kinds of veterans, inferences based on its data could be biased. BIRLS was searched for a record of each member of the combined study cohorts. Not all individuals were found: 23.4 percent of the participants and 24.8 percent of the referents were not found in BIRLS.

A veteran might not be found in BIRLS for varied reasons: (1) the record existed, but MFUA submitted insufficient information, such as a misspelled name, to identify it; (2) the requesting information was correct, but the BIRLS record includes a misspelling; (3) a veteran was not entered into BIRLS because the veteran or a surviving dependent had filed no claim for medical, educational, loan, death, or other benefits. Similarly, a claims folder—identified by BIRLS— might not be found because (1) the request went to the wrong VA regional office (VARO), (2) misfiling had occurred, (3) the file was transferred to another VARO, or (4) the file was transferred to a regional archives center. Finally a claims folder may be found but not contain the death certificate, the cause of death, or a legible copy of the certificate. For these reasons, we sought corroboration of fact of death from other sources.

TABLE 8-2. Vital Status Data as of December 31, 1996: Process and Availability

	Participants (n = 68,168)			Referents (n = 64,781)			Total (n = 132,949)		
	No.	% of Cohort	% of Dead	No.	% of Cohort	% of Dead	No.	% of Cohort	% of Dead
Not dead									
BIRLS record does not indicate death	32,684	47.9	—	30,172	46.6	—	62,856	47.3	—
No BIRLS record	15,975	23.4	—	16,063	24.8	32,038	24.1	—	
Death date after 12/31/96 (study cutoff)	992	1.5	—	873	1.3	—	1,865	1.4	—
Dead									
BIRLS-indicated death	18,345	26.9	99.1	17,487	27.0	98.9	35,832	27.0	99.0
BIRLS-indicated record at federal archives	172	0.3	1.0	186	0.3	1.1	358	0.3	1.0
Total		100.0	100.1		100.0	100.0		100.1	100.0

NOTE: BIRLS = Beneficiary Identification and Records Locator Subsystem.

Since 1979, the National Death Index (NDI), maintained by the National Center for Health Statistics, has assembled death certificate-derived mortality data from each of the 50 U.S. states, New York City, and the District of Columbia, as well as U.S. territories and protectorates. We first requested information on two 500-member samples of the participant and referent cohorts that had BIRLS records both without indication of death and with a BIRLS-noted Social Security number (SSN). Requiring an SSN allows for an efficient search within NDI and a check that the person identified in NDI is the same person in the study population.

NDI identified as dead 1.4 percent of the not-known-dead participant cohort sample and 1.8 percent of the not-known-dead referent cohort sample. These two rates were not statistically different ($p = .61$). Applying these rates to all of the not-known-dead individuals with BIRLS-noted Social Security numbers (21,513 participants and 16,917 referents), we estimate that 301 participant cohort deaths and 305 referent cohort deaths were not identified using the BIRLS procedures. These additions would increase the BIRLS-based study mortality rate from 27.2 to 27.7 percent (participants, from 27.2 to 27.6%; referents, from 27.3 to 27.8%).

However, we do not have SSNs for a large portion of the study population. In the two cohorts, of those not-known-dead, approximately 41 percent of the participants and 63 percent of the referents do not have any SSN in our database. The participant data that the Defense Threat Reduction Agency provided for this study from the Nuclear Test Personnel Review (NTPR) Program database include SSNs for some of the participant cohort who did not have SSNs listed in the BIRLS database. This NTPR source of information was not available for the referent cohort. Because using NTPR Social Security numbers would increase the likelihood of finding only participants in NDI, the study design excluded use of NTPR Social Security numbers because they would have allowed non-equivalent mortality ascertainment procedures for the two cohorts, introducing a bias into the ascertainment of the outcome data. However, the availability of NTPR Social Security numbers for participants did allow us to estimate how many deaths might have been ascertained if we had more complete SSN coverage. Thus, we submitted two additional 500-member samples of not-known-dead participants with NTPR SSNs to NDI. One group was in the BIRLS database without a BIRLS-noted SSN and one group was not in the BIRLS database at all. Because both BIRLS identification and SSN availability are associated with both vital status and the ascertainment of vital status, we wanted to use these samples to estimate the size of any differential in mortality rates that might stem from differences in information ascertainment rather than an effect of participation. Although these estimates were not used to adjust the analysis, they are useful in discussing the extent to which deaths have been missed and imbalanced ascertainment could influence study findings.

NDI identified as dead 4.6 percent of the not-known-dead participant cohort sample that was found in BIRLS without a BIRLS-noted SSN and 5.6 percent of the not-known-dead participant cohort sample that was not found in the BIRLS database at all.

Although ascertainment was not complete, these estimates provide a not-so-alarming approximation of the underascertainment of deaths in this study. There are 3,957 participants in the first group and 2,896 in the second. Applying the 4.6 and 5.6 percent sample estimates to the full groups would yield 182 deaths in the first group and 162 in the second. Applying these same rates to the participants without NTPR (or BIRLS) SSNs, we estimate an additional 411 deaths among the participants in BIRLS with neither BIRLS nor NTPR SSNs and 593 deaths among the participants with no record in BIRLS and no NTPR SSNs. Adding all of these groups together, we estimate that BIRLS did not identify 1,649 deaths. Therefore, the estimated BIRLS ascertainment rate for participants is 91.8 percent.

For the referent cohort, which does not have NTPR SSNs at all, we must use participant data to produce ascertainment estimates. Applying the 4.6 percent additional death ascertainment to referents in BIRLS but without a SSN yields 609 deaths; 5.6 percent additional deaths among referents not in BIRLS at all amounts to 900 deaths. Taken together, an estimated 1,814 referent cohort deaths were not ascertained by the BIRLS procedure, yielding an ascertainment of 90.7 percent of the deaths in the referent cohort.

Relatively few formal studies have been undertaken to determine the completeness of veteran death reporting via the BIRLS system, most of them involving either World War II or Vietnam era veterans. Studies of deaths among World War II veterans (Page, 1992; Page et al., 1995) estimated, respectively, that 92 and 95 percent of veteran deaths could be found in BIRLS. Studies of deaths among Vietnam era veterans (Page, 1993; Page et al., 1996) generally showed slightly lower percentages of BIRLS completeness, 90 percent, except that Boyle and Decoufle (1990) found BIRLS to be only 80 percent complete. A study by Fisher et al. (1995) of a group of hospitalized, largely pre-Vietnam-era veterans showed that BIRLS was 96 percent complete for death ascertainment. Although the methods employed across these studies are varied, all except the Boyle and Decoufle study showed the completeness of veteran death reporting in BIRLS to be 90–95 percent. Although the veterans studied here are, for the most part, neither World War II nor Vietnam era vets, we believe that the completeness of death reporting in BIRLS is roughly the same among the veterans in the present study.

DATE OF DEATH

BIRLS was the principal source of death date for the study analyses (see Table 8-3). An actual date was noted for 97.2 percent of the known dead individuals. No date of death was identified for less than 0.1 percent of the known deaths. Another 2.1 percent of the death dates were obtained from the VA Master Index, the death certificate, or NDI. For most of the remaining deaths, we were able to calculate an approximate date of death based on the date a record was transferred from a VA regional office to a federal archives center. This estimate is possible because VA sends to the archives only those VA benefit claims records that are inactive due to the death of veteran and any surviving beneficiaries.

TABLE 8-3. Date-of-Death Data: Process and Availability—Deaths Only

	Participants with Death Indicated (*n* = 18,517)		Referents with Death Indicated (*n* = 17,673)		Total with Death Indicated (*n* = 36,190)	
Date-of-Death Source	No.	%	No.	%	No.	%
VA BIRLS	18,120	97.9	17,063	96.6	35,183	97.2
VA Master Index	77	0.4	291	1.6	368	1.0
Death certificate	236	1.3	163	0.9	399	1.1
National Death Index	1	0.0	0	—	1	0.0
Imputed (using date of claims folder transfer to the federal archives)	64	0.4	140	0.8	204	0.6
Problem or missing	19	0.1	16	0.1	35	0.1

NOTE: BIRLS = Beneficiary Identification and Records Locator Subsystem; VA = Department of Veterans Affairs.

We used the records with both a BIRLS-noted date of death and a date of folder transfer to archives to calculate the lag time between death and record transfer. Because the efficiency of both the VA and the National Archives and Records Administration (NARA) may have varied over the years, we calculated these lags by year. These lags, generalized to multiyear periods as appropriate, were then applied to the 204 records that had only the record transfer date to impute a date of death.

CAUSE-OF-DEATH ACQUISITION

The two sources of cause-of-death information are both death certificate based: the death certificate itself and electronic tapes compiled from the death certificates. The BIRLS database provides the location of the claims folder: a specific VA regional office (VARO) or a specific federal archives center (FARC). Following established VA and NARA procedures, we requested that the VARO and archives staff pull the folder and send us a copy of the death certificate for each death. Our contract nosologist supplied codes for all causes of death listed and selected one as the underlying cause and the others, if any, as associated causes.

In cases in which the VAROs and FARCs could not produce a death certificate and for which we had date of death, we requested death certificate information from NDI-Plus if the death occurred in 1979 or later. NDI-Plus returned an electronic tape with identifying information and underlying and associated causes of death.

Table 8-4 and Table 8-5 are limited to those members of the study population who are known to have died (excluding those who died after December 31, 1996). Of these 36,190 individuals, a cause of death is not available for 5.9 percent. The difference between the participant cohort's 4.5 percent and the referent cohort's 7.3 percent is statistically significant. For the causes of death that we did obtain, 65.5 percent came from the death certificate and 34.5 percent from the National Death Index-Plus.

CAUSE-OF-DEATH VALIDATION

To determine the level of agreement between the two sources of cause-of-death codes, we processed a sample of 200 records through both ascertainment paths. Neither source—the contract nosologist or the NDI-Plus database—was considered the standard; discrepancies were counted, not correct and incorrect codes. Eleven of the underlying cause-of-death codes were sufficiently different so that the death would be assigned to a different cause-specific analysis group. (Another 10 had differences [e.g., in the fourth digit of the International Classification of Diseases code] that exceeded the level of detail examined in this report.) For 4 of the 11, the two sources had the same codes but specified different ones as the underlying cause of death.

TABLE 8-4. Cause-of-Death Availability—Deaths Only

	Participants with Death Indicated		Referents with Death Indicated		Total with Death Indicated	
Availability	No.	%	No.	%	No.	%
Available	17,675	95.5	16,378	92.7	34,053	94.1
Missing	842	4.5	1,295	7.3	2,137	5.9
Total	18,517	100.0	17,673	100.0	36,190	100.0

TABLE 8-5. Cause-of-Death Source—Deaths Only

	Participants with Death Indicated		Referents with Death Indicated		Total with Death Indicated	
Source	No.	%	No.	%	No.	%
Death certificate	11,893	67.3	10,422	63.6	22,315	65.5
NDI-Plus	5,782	32.7	5,956	36.4	11,738	34.5
Total	18,517	100.0	16,378	100.0	34,053	100.0

NOTE: NDI = National Death Index.

We looked at the records that had a malignant neoplasm in any of the cause fields from either source to determine whether cancers—the prime endpoint of this study—were noted similarly by the two coding sources. There were 74 records with malignancy codes; of these, 6 were discrepant in the underlying cause-of-death field. Five of these involved the selection of the underlying cause from among all listed causes. Of the six discrepancies, three do not affect the analysis of the broad category of all-malignancy deaths but, because they select a different site-specific cancer, would affect that level of analysis.

9

Analysis Structure

OVERVIEW

The analysis plan for the Five Series Study was structured to check data validity, test hypotheses, and interactively explore data to follow leads arising from data analysis. The study was designed to address whether

- participation in at least one of the five selected atmospheric nuclear weapons tests is associated with increased mortality hazard; and
- participants who were more likely to have been highly exposed to radiation would have increased mortality hazard relative to participants who were less likely to have been highly exposed.

The basic comparison involves the survival experience of participants relative to that of referent cohort members. Because various diseases have different degrees of radiogenicity (Mettler and Upton, 1995), hazard ratios have been calculated for mortality from all causes, all malignancies, and leukemia (excluding chronic lymphocytic leukemia). Other radiogenic cancers, along with a selection of presumed nonradiogenic diseases and conditions, are also examined. Disease categories were discussed and defined, using *International Classification of Diseases,* 9th Edition, codes, before analysis began (see below).

AVAILABLE DATA

Data available for the analysis of survival times consist of measures or indicators of (1) presumed radiation exposure, (2) individual and military service characteristics that might confound an association between exposure and outcome, and (3) mortality outcome. Table 9-1 presents the variables that were included in the analysis dataset. It should be noted that variables were not all of the same quality with regard to completeness and validity.

TABLE 9-1. Variables Considered for Analysis and Their Utility

Variable	Example	Utility[a]
Participant status	Participant	+
Sex	Male	–
Paygrade	E3	+
Branch of service	Air Force, Army, Marines, Navy	+
Selection series	CASTLE	+
Date of selection series[b]	April 1, 1953	+
Location	Pacific	+
Shot	BRAVO	–
Number of series	3	+
Number of shots	12	–
Unit category[c]	Technical	+
Unit of assignment	9740 TSU Chemical Section	+
Rank/rating	Private, PVT2	–
Occupation	E.g., pilot, navigator	–
Tasks during test	Cloud sampler pilot	–
Dose	2.4 rem	–
Device	Thermonuclear	–
Date of birth	January 15, 1923	+
Vital status	Dead	+[e]
Date of death	March 7, 1972	+[d,e]
Age at selection series[d]	Date of selection series minus date of birth	+
Years since atomic test exposure[d]	Date of death or censoring minus date of selection series	+/–[e]
Age at death or censure[d]	Date of death or censoring minus date of birth	+/–[e]
Calendar decade of death[d]	1960s	+/–[e]
Decade since selection series[d]	20–30 years since shot	+/–[e]
Underlying cause of death	Malignant neoplasm of the lung	+
Associated causes of death	Hypertensive heart disease	+

[a] Plus or minus assigned based on general consideration of validity and completeness; a plus indicates that data are available and of good quality; a minus indicates that data are either unavailable or of poor quality.
[b] The first day of the operational period of the selection series.
[c] Categories created and assigned based on unit of assignment.
[d] Value calculated from specified dates in dataset.
[e] Quality of fact and date data is discussed in this report. For known deaths, the quality is excellent; the Department of Veterans Affairs data system may not have ascertained all deaths of study cohort members.

ANALYSIS

Variables

The variables included in the basic analyses are participant status, age at selection series, paygrade, branch of service, and selection series. Analyses also explore relationships using variables such as land versus sea series; age–calendar time; disease latency; series and *post-series* time periods; number of series; and associated causes of death. (The definitions and rationale for the use of these variables are described elsewhere in this report.)

To appropriately test the second question—whether a dose–response relationship exists between radiation exposure and mortality hazard—an at-least-ordinal variable that ranks an exposure surrogate measure would be needed. (Note: A working group of the committee overseeing the Five Series Study has reported [IOM, 1995; reprinted in Appendix A of this report] that the extensive dosimetry categorization and reconstruction data developed by the Nuclear Test Personnel Review Program of the Defense Threat Reduction Agency* are not suitable for use in epidemiologic investigations of dose–response. This analysis plan does not, therefore, use the dosimetry data as exposure variables in the statistical analysis.) These surrogates could incorporate information—from military records, eyewitness accounts, and historical records—known about groups more and less likely to have received higher radiation doses. Using the exposure surrogates, statistical models could test for these proxy dose–response relationships. (See Chapter 7.)

Type of Analysis

The research group defined two analytic approaches. The first uses standardized mortality ratios (SMRs), calculated for each cohort (participant and referent) separately using standard rates adjusted for age and time distributions (Marsh et al., 1998; Rothman and Greenland, 1998.). The second involves proportional hazards modeling using the wider range of available covariates (Allison, 1995).

SMRs are a commonly used tool to compare death rates among a cohort of interest to those in a larger, reference population, customarily the U.S. general population. The deaths that actually occur in the cohort of interest are labeled “observed” deaths; one also calculates the “expected” number of deaths that would have occurred had the members of the cohort died at the same rate as the U.S. population with the same age, race, and sex distribution. The ratio of observed to expected deaths is an SMR, which is equal to 1.0 if the number of

*The organizational locus of the Nuclear Test Personnel Review Program within the Department of Defense has been the Defense Nuclear Agency (until June 1996), the Defense Special Weapons Agency (until October 1998), and, currently, the Defense Threat Reduction Agency.

deaths observed in the cohort of interest is the same as the number of deaths expected to have occurred if the cohort members had died at U.S. population death rates.

Sex and race information was not included in the datasets for this study. For the 61.7 percent of deaths for which we were able to acquire death certificates, race and sex information is available. Less than half a percent (0.4%) of the death certificates were coded as female; between 8 and 9 percent as black. These proportions may not accurately reflect the unknown percentages of male and black members of the participant and referent cohorts. Because both race and sex are associated with mortality (both survival time and cause of death), they do not provide valid estimates of the full at-risk cohort. We used white male population rates for SMR calculations.

SMRs thus show whether the mortality of the cohort of interest is higher or lower than that of the U.S. population. One typically sees SMRs for veterans cohorts that are less than 1.0. Reasons given focus on the requirement that military servicemen pass an entrance physical and also pass periodic physical fitness exams while in military service, both effectively screening in favor of healthier individuals versus their general civilian counterparts. Not only is this healthiness thought to produce lower death rates among active duty military personnel, but lower mortality rates apparently persist even after discharge from active duty (Seltzer and Jablon, 1974, 1977). Such effects seen among occupational groups have been labeled the "healthy worker effect," and by analogy, lower SMRs among military veterans can be attributed to a "healthy soldier effect." Despite this limitation, SMRs provide a way to compare the mortality of the cohort of interest to that of the general population. Also, because SMRs are based on standard distributions of deaths, they can be compared across studies. We used OCMAP Plus software to compute SMRs (Marsh et al., 1998).

Cox proportional hazard ratio analysis (Cox, 1972) is used for the core analyses in this report. We implemented these analyses using the SAS program PHREG (SAS Institute, 1996). In this approach, the risk of death—in statistical terms, the *hazard*—is modeled in a regression that includes a baseline hazard as well as coefficients that represent the additional hazards associated with various factors such as—in this case—nuclear test series participation. The coefficient associated with a factor represents a hazard ratio, which can be interpreted as a relative risk of death that remains constant over the follow-up period. In our analyses, coefficients were included for test series participation, age at time of first participation, and age at time of first participation squared and cubed. Hazard ratios are considered statistically significant if their associated 95 percent confidence interval excludes the value 1.0. The time scale for these models was attained age, which is thought to be the most appropriate scale for the kinds of analyses we undertook (Korn et al., 1997).

Rather than fashion regression models that included risk estimates for other factors such as test series, branch of service, and paygrade, we chose to include these as stratification variables. Although this choice does not permit the estimation of risks associated with the stratification variables, it does allow more complete control of the effects of these variables (see Allison [1995] for further detail). Finally, if we did not have definitive evidence of death for an individual, he was considered to be *not known dead* (alive); if the individual was thought to be dead, but there was no date of death or date of birth (there were only 38 of these), this record was excluded from the analyses.

Diagnosis Groups

Based on tables from other studies of atomic veterans (e.g., Pearce et al., 1997) yet expanded, the staff and committee chose which categories of diagnosis codes to examine: (1) the broad categories of noncancer causes of death; (2) all malignant neoplasms; and (3) focused groups of malignancies, including leukemias and other putatively radiogenic malignancies. Table 9-2 and Table 9-3 present the cause-of-death categories considered in this report.

TABLE 9-2. Broad Categories of Noncancer Causes of Death as Grouped by ICD-9 Codes

Broad Category	ICD-9 Code
Infectious and parasitic diseases	001–139
Benign neoplasms	210–239
Endocrine, nutritional, and metabolic diseases and immunity disorders	240–279
Diseases of the blood and blood-forming organs	280–289
Mental disorders	290–319
Diseases of the nervous system and sense organs	320–389
Circulatory disease	390–459
Respiratory disease	460–519
Digestive disease	520–579
Diseases of the genitourinary system	580–629
Diseases of the skin and subcutaneous tissue	680–709
Diseases of the musculoskeletal system and connective tissue	710–739
Congenital anomalies	740–759
Symptoms, signs, and ill-defined conditions	780–799
All external causes	800–999
Total*	001–139, 210–999

*Not included are complications of pregnancy, childbirth, and the puerperium, and certain conditions originating in the perinatal period.

SOURCE: *International Classification of Diseases,* 9th Edition (ICD-9) (USDHHS, 1991).

TABLE 9-3. Cause-of-Death Categories Within Broad Category of Malignant Neoplasms

Site ICD-9	Code
Lip, oral cavity, and pharynx	140–149
Digestive organs and peritoneum	
Esophagus	150
Stomach	151
Small intestine	152
Colon	153
Rectum	154
Liver and intrahepatic bile ducts	155
Gallbladder	156
Pancreas	157
Respiratory and intrathoracic organs	
Nasal	160
Larynx	161
Lung	162
Bone, connective tissue, skin, and breast	
Bone	170
Connective tissue	171
Skin	172
Skin—nonmelanoma	173
Breast	
Genitourinary organs	
Prostate	185
Testis	186
Bladder	188
Kidney	189
Other	
Brain and nervous system	191, 192
Thyroid	193
Other solid cancer	140–199
Total hematological	200–208
Non-Hodgkin's lymphoma	200, 202
Hodgkin's disease	201
Multiple myeloma	203
Leukemia	204–208
Leukemia, excluding chronic lymphoid leukemia	204.0, 204.2–208.9
Total*	140–208

*Not listed separately are malignant neoplasms of the retroperitoneum and peritoneum; other digestive organs; pleura; thymus, heart, and mediastinum; other respiratory and intrathoracic organs; female breast; female genital organs; penis and other male genital organs; eye; other (than thyroid) endocrine glands; other, ill-defined, secondary, and unspecified sites.

SOURCE: *International Classification of Diseases,* 9th Edition (ICD-9) (USDHHS, 1991).

10

Description of Cohort Characteristics

Table 10-1, Table 10-2, Table 10-3, Table 10-4, Table 10-5 through Table 10-6 display characteristics of the participant and referent groups, separately and combined. Based on the cohort selection protocols described in Chapter 4 and Chapter 5, the study population for this report consists of 68,168 veterans who participated in at least one of the five nuclear test series selected for this study and 64,781 veterans who served at the same time but did not participate in any nuclear test. As previously discussed in Chapter 9, race and sex data were not available for the individuals studied. By selecting a referent cohort with similar distribution of other characteristics—such as age, branch of service, time of service, paygrade, and type of military unit—we think that the race and sex distributions should be approximately equivalent. Table 10-1 shows the distribution by branch of service; Table 10-2, selection series. Service and series noted are both at the time warranting selection into the study (i.e., for participants, status at time of first participation in one of the five series; for referents, status at time coinciding with selection relative to the corresponding participant).

The age variables, displayed in Table 10-3 and Table 10-4, all derive from the date of birth for an individual at the start date of the selection series. Typical of an active-duty military population, 63 percent of these cohorts are less than 26 years of age and 87 percent are less than 36 years of age. The set of identification files from the contractor that prepared the lists of test participants eligible for this study was the major source of birth dates for the participant cohort, followed by VA databases. Such information was not available for members of the referent cohort; VA data were the primary sources for them.

Table 10-5 shows the distribution of military paygrade at the time of selection series participation. The paygrade groupings used in the study analysis are aggregations of the 23 separate potential paygrades (see Appendix E for details). The group of missing paygrades is coded separately because of unknown characteristics that might modify these individuals' risks in indeterminable ways.

Table 10-6 displays the distribution of participant and referent cohort members across branch of service and selection series.

TABLE 10-1. Cohort Member Characteristics: Branch of Military Service

	Participants (n = 68,168)		Referents (n = 64,781)		Total (n = 132,949)	
Service	No.	%	No.	%	No.	%
Air Force	12,865	18.9	11,904	18.4	24,769	18.6
Army	26,082	38.3	24,992	38.6	51,074	38.4
Marines	5,000	7.3	4,865	7.5	9,865	7.4
Navy	24,221	35.5	23,020	35.5	47,241	35.5

TABLE 10-2. Cohort Member Characteristics: Selection Series

	Participants (n = 68,168)		Referents (n = 64,781)		Total (n = 132,949)	
Selection Series	No.	%	No.	%	No.	%
GREENHOUSE (1951)	9,528	14.0	9,146	14.1	18,674	14.0
UPSHOT-KNOTHOLE (1953)	18,473	27.1	17,776	27.4	36,249	27.3
CASTLE (1954)	15,685	23.0	15,221	23.5	30,906	23.2
REDWING (1956)	12,923	19.0	12,627	19.5	25,550	19.2
PLUMBBOB (1957)	11,559	17.0	10,011	15.5	21,570	16.2

TABLE 10-3. Cohort Member Characteristics: Age at Start of Follow-Up

	Participants (n = 68,168)		Referents (n = 64,781)		Total (n = 132,949)	
Age	No.	%	No.	%	No.	%
<26	42,972	63.0	41,131	63.5	84,103	63.3
≥ 26 and <36	16,352	24.0	15,802	24.4	32,154	24.2
≥ 36 and <46	7,280	10.7	6,433	9.9	13,713	10.3
≥ 46 and <56	1,421	2.1	1,259	1.9	2,680	2.0
≥ 56 and <66	137	0.2	152	0.2	289	0.2
≥ 66	2	0.0	4	0.0	6	0.0
Missing	4	0.0	0	—	4	0.0

TABLE 10-4. Cohort Member Characteristics: Source of Date of Birth

	Participants (n = 68,168)		Referents (n = 64,781)		Total (n = 132,949)	
Source	No.	%	No.	%	No.	%
VA Beneficiary Identification and Records Locator Subsystem	8,576	12.6	30,983	47.8	39,559	29.8
Imputed (using service, series, and paygrade groupings)	2,896	4.3	5,953	9.2	8,849	6.7
JAYCOR (Department of Defense contractor)	45,216	66.3	0	—	45,216	34.0
Military personnel records (National Personnel Records Center, St. Louis)	1,569	2.3	4,282	6.6	5,851	4.4
VA Master Index (pre-1972)	9,908	14.5	23,563	36.4	33,471	25.2
Missing and unimputable (missing paygrade also)	3	0.0	0	—	3	0.0

NOTE: VA = Department of Veterans Affairs.

TABLE 10-5. Cohort Member Characteristics: Paygrade

	Participants (*n* = 68,168)		Referents (*n* = 64,781)		Total (*n* = 132,949)	
Paygrade Groupings	No.	%	No.	%	No.	%
E1–E3, junior enlisted	25,067	36.8	24,761	38.2	49,828	37.5
E4–E5, midlevel enlisted	20,141	29.6	19,800	30.6	39,941	30.0
E6–E9, senior enlisted	8,223	12.1	7,946	12.3	16,169	12.2
W1–W4, warrant officer	571	0.8	429	0.7	1,000	0.8
O1–O3, company officer	7,285	10.7	7,632	11.8	14,917	11.2
O4–O6, field officer	6,075	8.9	4,139	6.4	10,214	7.7
O7–O10, general officer	333	0.5	62	0.1	395	0.3
Missing	473	0.7	12	0.0	485	0.4

TABLE 10-6. Distribution of Participant and Referent Cohort Members by Branch of Service and Selection Series

	Selection Series											
	GREENHOUSE		UPSHOT-KNOTHOLE		CASTLE		REDWING		PLUMBBOB		Five Series Total	
Service	Participants No. (%)	Referents No. (%)	Participants No. (%)	Referents No. (%)	Participants No. (%)	Referents No. (%)	Participants No. (%)	Referents No. (%)	Participants No. (%)	Referents No. (%)	Participants No. (%)	Referents No. (%)
Air Force	2,847	2,771	2,353	1,764	2,631	2,588	3,019	2,981	2,015	1,800	12,865	11,904
	(29.9)	(30.0)	(12.7)	(9.9)	(16.8)	(17.0)	(23.4)	(23.6)	(17.4)	(18.0)	(18.9)	(18.4)
Army	2,218	2,193	13,145	13,358	1,525	1,512	2,147	2,126	7,047	5,803	26,082	24,992
	(23.3)	(24.0)	(71.2)	(75.1)	(9.7)	(9.9)	(16.6)	(16.8)	(61.0)	(58.0)	(38.3)	(38.6)
Marines	76	69	2,262	2,175	297	290	245	238	2,120	2,093	5,000	4,865
	(0.8)	(0.8)	(12.2)	(12.2)	(1.9)	(1.9)	(1.9)	(1.9)	(18.3)	(20.9)	(7.3)	(7.5)
Navy	4,387	4,113	713	479	11,232	10,831	7,512	7,282	377	315	24,221	23,020
	(46.0)	(45.0)	(3.9)	(2.7)	(71.6)	(71.2)	(58.1)	(57.7)	(3.3)	(3.1)	(35.5)	(35.5)
Total	9,528	9,146	18,473	17,776	15,685	15,221	12,923	12,627	11,559	10,011	68,168	64,781
	(100.0)	(100.0)	(100.0)	(100.0)	(100.0)	(100.0)	(100.0)	(100.0)	(100.0)	(100.0)	(100.0)	(100.0)

11

Findings

In this chapter, we present the findings from our standardized mortality ratio and proportional hazards analyses.[1] We begin with tests of the primary study endpoints and the presentation of some descriptive data. The findings from these analyses suggested additional avenues of investigation, the results of which are then reported.

TESTS OF PREDETERMINED PRINCIPAL ENDPOINTS

We had determined in advance of data collection that participant versus referent mortality rates would be formally compared for three endpoints—all causes, all malignancies, and all leukemia minus chronic lymphoid leukemia (CLL). We had further decided to examine these outcomes using both standardized mortality ratios (SMRs) and proportional hazards analyses. SMRs were used to compare mortality rates for participant and referent subjects with U.S. white male population rates.[2] However, these SMRs take into account only age and calendar year of death, and the mortality rates of the U.S. general population are generally higher than those of military veterans. When a comparable referent group is available, proportional hazards analyses allow for simultaneous control of design variables (via stratification) as well as tighter control for age differences (via covariate adjustment) and thus provide a better basis for estimating the difference in mortality experience of the two groups.

SMR data in Table 11-1 show that the SMRs for both all-cause mortality and all-malignancy mortality were almost equal for participants and referents, whereas participants had a higher SMR for leukemia death (0.75) than did refer

[1] See Chapter 9 and Appendix C for explanation of these methods.

[2] See Chapter 9 for discussion of the use of white male rates.

ents (0.65). As anticipated, all SMRs are less than 1.00, indicating that both the participant and the referent cohorts had lower mortality than the general population—the "healthy veteran effect" (Seltzer and Jablon, 1974, 1977). The proportional hazards analyses also show—with estimated hazard ratios (HRs)—that participants and referents were at similar risk of all-cause mortality (HR = 1.00) and all-malignancy mortality (HR = 1.02), and participants had an estimated 14 percent higher risk of leukemia death (HR = 1.14). However, none of these hazard ratios is significantly different from 1.00, indicating that there were no statistically significant differences between the participant and referent cohorts on these outcome measures.

DESCRIPTIVE ANALYSES OF PREDETERMINED ADDITIONAL MORTALITY ENDPOINTS

We also looked at a number of mortality endpoints that had been examined in other studies, particularly cancer endpoints. Table 11-2 shows SMRs for broad categories of noncancer causes of death. Only one SMR was greater than 1.00—symptoms, signs, and ill-defined conditions. Proportional hazards analysis shows only two significant differences. Participants had a significantly higher risk of death due to external causes (1.08; 95% CI 1.02–1.16) and a significantly lower risk of death due to unknown cause (0.62; 95% CI 0.57–0.67). The latter is not surprising because it reflects the fact that the causes were missing for 4.5 percent of participant deaths versus 7.3 percent of referent deaths, a statistically significant difference (see Table 8-4 and related discussion). Participants also had higher risks of death due to diseases of the musculoskeletal system (1.43; 95% CI 0.86–2.38) and congenital anomalies (1.59; 95% CI 0.72– 3.51); however, these are based on relatively small numbers of deaths.

Table 11-3 shows data for various cancer mortality endpoints in some detail. Again, almost all SMRs are less than 1.00. The six cancer sites with estimated hazard ratios greater than 1.2 are nasal cancer (2.64; 95% CI 1.02–6.82), thyroid cancer (2.33; 95% CI 0.83–6.55), cancer of the testes (1.62; 95% CI 0.59–4.46), male breast cancer (1.39; 95% CI 0.53–3.66), bone cancer (1.21; 95% CI 0.57–2.60), and prostate cancer (1.20; 95% CI 1.03–1.40). Only the risks of death due to nasal cancer and prostate cancer were significantly higher among participants than referents. Among the hematologic cancers, the risks for all leukemia (1.15; 95% CI 0.93–1.43) and leukemia minus chronic lymphoid leukemia (CLL) (1.14; 95% CI 0.90–1.44) were both elevated, albeit not significantly, among participants.

Table 11-4 shows a more detailed breakdown of leukemia deaths by sub-type, as available from death certificates. The highest hazard ratios are associated with two types of acute leukemia: lymphoid leukemia excluding CLL (2.05; 95% CI 0.71–5.92) and myeloid leukemia excluding chronic myeloid leukemia (1.44; 95% CI 1.00–2.09).

TABLE 11-1. Number of Observed Deaths and Standardized Mortality Ratio (SMR), by Cohort, and Hazard Ratio for Participants Relative to Referents—for Planned Analysis Causes of Death

		Participant Cohort		Referent Cohort		
Hypothesized Categories	ICD-9 Codes	Observed Deaths	SMR[b]	Observed Deaths	SMR[b]	Hazard Ratio[a] (95% CI)
All causes	001–799, E800–E999	18,498	0.71	17,657	0.73	1.00 (0.98–1.02)
All malignancies	140–208	5,081	0.74	4,702	0.74	1.02 (0.98–1.06)
All leukemias	204–208	185	0.74	149	0.64	1.15 (0.93–1.43)
Leukemias (minus chronic lymphoid leukemia)	204.0, 204.2–208.9	156	0.75	126	0.65	1.14 (0.90–1.44)

NOTE: CI = confidence interval; ICD-9 = *International Classification of Diseases,* 9th Edition.

[a] Participant cohort relative to referent cohort. Proportional hazards model controls for series, service, and paygrade by stratification and age by covariate adjustment.

[b] SMRs calculated using the OCMAP program and U.S. rates for white males.

TABLE 11-2. Number of Observed Deaths and Standardized Mortality Ratio (SMR), by Cohort, and Hazard Ratio for Participants Relative to Referents—for Broad Cause-of-Death Categories

		Participant Cohort		Referent Cohort		
Broad Cause of Death Category	ICD-9 Codes	Observed Deaths	SMR[b]	Observed Deaths	SMR[b]	Hazard Ratio[a] (95% CI)
Infectious and parasitic diseases	001–139	177	0.57	186	0.64	0.92 (0.75–1.13)
Malignant neoplasms	140–208	5,081	0.74	4,702	0.74	1.02 (0.98–1.06)
Benign neoplasms, carcinoma in situ, and neoplasms of uncertain behavior	210–239	57	0.68	58	0.75	0.86 (0.60–1.25)
Endocrine, nutritional, and metabolic diseases, and immunity disorders	240–279	311	0.54	293	0.55	1.02 (0.87–1.20)
Diseases of the blood and blood-forming organs	280–289	46	0.61	43	0.63	0.98 (0.64–1.50)
Mental disorders	290–319	166	0.73	143	0.68	1.09 (0.87–1.37)
Diseases of the nervous system and sense organs	320–389	225	0.51	214	0.52	0.96 (0.79–1.16)
Diseases of the circulatory system	390–459	6,970	0.62	6,487	0.63	1.02 (0.99–1.06)
Diseases of the respiratory system	460–519	1,151	0.63	1,043	0.63	1.06 (0.97–1.15)
Diseases of the digestive system	520–579	956	0.77	891	0.77	1.04 (0.95–1.14)
Diseases of the genitourinary system	580–629	173	0.57	168	0.61	0.98 (0.79–1.22)

Diseases of the skin and subcutaneous tissue	680–709	13	0.66	17	0.96	0.78 (0.38–1.62)
Diseases of the musculoskeletal system and connective tissue	710–739	39	0.76	25	0.53	1.43 (0.86–2.38)
Congenital anomalies	740–759	16	0.27	10	0.18	1.59 (0.72–3.51)
Symptoms, signs, and ill-defined conditions	780–799	289	1.08	320	1.28	0.88 (0.75–1.03)
External causes of injury and poisoning	E800–E999	2,004	0.76	1,771	0.71	1.08 (1.02–1.16)
Unknown cause[c]		842		1,295		0.62 (0.57–0.67)
Total		18,498	0.71	17,657	0.73	1.00 (0.98–1.02)

NOTE: CI = confidence interval; ICD-9 = *International Classification of Diseases,* 9th Edition.

[a]Participant cohort relative to referent cohort. Proportional hazards model controls for series, service, and paygrade by stratification and age by covariate adjustment.
[b]SMRs calculated using the OCMAP program and U.S. rates for white males.
[c]Known dead with unknown cause.

TABLE 11-3. Number of Observed Deaths and Standardized Mortality Ratio (SMR), by Cohort, and Hazard Ratio for Participants Relative to Referents—for Causes of Death Within the Broad Category of Malignant Neoplasms

		Participant Cohort		Referent Cohort		
Malignant Neoplasm Cause of Death	ICD-9 Codes	Observed Deaths	SMR[b]	Observed Deaths	SMR[b]	Hazard Ratio[a] (95% CI)
Lip, oral cavity, and pharynx	140–149	148	0.85	142	0.88	0.99 (0.79–1.25)
Salivary gland	142	10	0.89	8	0.77	1.07 (0.42–2.75)
Digestive organs and peritoneum	150–159	1,114	0.69	1,073	0.71	0.99 (0.91–1.07)
Esophagus	150	153	0.84	154	0.91	0.92 (0.74–1.16)
Stomach	151	129	0.60	133	0.67	0.94 (0.74–1.20)
Small intestine	152	10	0.71	10	0.76	0.95 (0.39–2.30)
Colon	153	383	0.67	343	0.65	1.07 (0.92–1.24)
Rectum	154	72	0.56	75	0.63	0.91 (0.66–1.27)
Liver and intrahepatic bile ducts	155	93	0.77	90	0.81	0.98 (0.73–1.31)
Gallbladder	156	29	0.78	26	0.76	1.08 (0.63–1.83)
Pancreas	157	222	0.67	227	0.74	0.91 (0.76–1.10)
Respiratory and intrathoracic organs	160–165	1,927	0.73	1,860	0.76	0.99 (0.93–1.06)
Nasal	160	15	1.64	6	0.70	2.64 (1.02–6.82)
Larynx	161	74	0.84	73	0.89	0.99 (0.72–1.37)
Trachea, bronchus, and lung	162	1,827	0.72	1,766	0.75	0.99 (0.93–1.06)
Bone, connective tissue, skin, and breast	170–176	183		168		1.01 (0.82–1.25)
Bone	170	15	0.83	12	0.71	1.21 (0.57–2.60)
Connective tissue	171	26	0.71	23	0.67	1.07 (0.61–1.88)
Skin—melanoma	172	101	0.82	90	0.78	1.02 (0.77–1.36)
Skin—nonmelanoma	173	30	0.88	25	0.79	1.14 (0.67–1.94)

Male breast[c]	175	10	1.23	7	0.93	1.39 (0.53–3.66)
Genitourinary organs	179–189	622	0.76	525	0.71	1.09 (0.97–1.23)
Prostate	185	387	0.85	295	0.72	1.20 (1.03–1.40)
Testis	186	10	0.41	6	0.26	1.62 (0.59–4.46)
Bladder	188	80	0.53	92	0.67	0.80 (0.59–1.09)
Kidney	189	136	0.73	127	0.73	1.00 (0.78–1.27)
Other and unspecified sites	190–199	618	0.94	530	0.87	1.10 (0.98–1.24)
Brain and other nervous system	191, 192	143	0.68	154	0.78	0.87 (0.69–1.09)
Thyroid	193	13	1.08	5	0.45	2.33 (0.83–6.55)
Lymphatic and hematopoietic tissue	200–208	469	0.71	404	0.66	1.09 (0.95–1.24)
Non-Hodgkin's lymphoma	200, 202	174	0.70	156	0.68	1.06 (0.85–1.32)
Hodgkin's disease	201	28	0.52	31	0.61	0.87 (0.52–1.45)
Multiple myeloma	203	82	0.80	68	0.72	1.10 (0.79–1.52)
Leukemia	204–208	185	0.74	149	0.64	1.15 (0.93–1.43)
Leukemia, excluding chronic lymphoid leukemia	204.0, 204.2–208.9	156	0.75	126	0.65	1.14 (0.90–1.44)
Total malignant neoplasm	140–208	5,081	0.74	4,702	0.74	1.02 (0.98–1.06)

NOTE: CI = confidence interval; ICD-9 = *International Classification of Diseases,* 9th Edition.

[a]Participant cohort relative to referent cohort. Proportional hazards model controls for series, service, and paygrade by stratification and age by covariate adjustment.
[b]SMRs calculated using the OCMAP program and U.S. rates for white males.
[c]In addition to the male breast cancer deaths counted in this table, there were 1 participant and 11 referent female breast cancer deaths.

TABLE 11-4. Number of Observed Deaths and Standardized Mortality Ratio (SMR), by Cohort, and Hazard Ratio for Participants Relative to Referents—for the ICD-9-Defined Subtypes of Leukemia

		Participant Cohort		Referent Cohort		
Cause of Death	ICD-9 Codes	Observed Deaths	SMR[b]	Observed Deaths	SMR[b]	Hazard Ratio[a] (95% CI)
Lymphoid leukemia	204	40	0.53	28	0.40	1.37 (0.84–2.22)
Lymphoid leukemia, excluding CLL	204.0, 204.2–204.9	11	0.39	5	0.19	2.05 (0.71–5.92)
CLL	204.1	29	0.59	23	0.51	1.22 (0.71–2.11)
Myeloid leukemia	205	101	0.82	75	0.66	1.24 (0.92–1.68)
Myeloid leukemia, excluding CML	205.0, 205.2–205.9	72	0.82	46	0.56	1.44 (1.00–2.09)
CML	205.1	29	0.77	29	0.82	0.92 (0.54–1.54)
Monocytic leukemia	206	2	0.49	3	0.80	0.67 (0.11–4.04)
Other specified leukemia	207	6	0.73	5	0.65	1.04 (0.31–3.47)
Leukemia of unspecified cell type	208	36	0.59	38	0.68	0.87 (0.55–1.38)
Total leukemia	204–208	185	0.74	149	0.64	1.15 (0.93–1.43)

NOTE: CI = confidence interval; CLL = chronic lymphoid leukemia; CML = chronic myeloid leukemia; and ICD-9 = *International Classification of Diseases*, 9th Edition.

[a] Participant cohort relative to referent cohort. Proportional hazards model controls for series, service, and paygrade by stratification and age by covariate adjustment.
[b] SMRs calculated using the OCMAP program and U.S. rates for white males.

INVESTIGATING LEUKEMIA RISK BY LAND AND SEA SERIES PARTICIPATION

We stated earlier that although we had not identified any unambiguous proxy measures for radiation dose, we had considered the possibility that the different test series or the land and sea series represent differences in exposure experience.

Exposures were not uniformly distributed within series. Operation PLUMBBOB, for example, consisted of 30 tests, including safety tests that produced negligible yields as well as detonations of up to 44 kt (Harris et al., 1981). A formal test of heterogeneity of leukemia minus CLL risks among the individual test series was not statistically significant ($\chi^2 = 7.191$, 4 df, $p = .13$); thus, we removed the series-specific analyses from the core presentation of this report. To be complete, however, risk estimates of individual test series, service branch, and paygrade groupings are presented in Appendix E.

Our interest in the land–sea dichotomy was based on the possibility that the exposure experience was qualitatively—and perhaps quantitatively—different at the two test sites. In Table 11-5, land series participation is defined as attendance at UPSHOT-KNOTHOLE, PLUMBBOB, or any other test series conducted at the Nevada Test Site, regardless of a participant's selection series. Similarly, attendance at GREENHOUSE, CASTLE, REDWING, or any other series conducted at the Pacific Proving Ground constituted sea series participation, regardless of selection series. Members of the referent cohort were classified only by their counterpart's selection series. Thus, because a participant may have attended both land and sea tests, the number of land series participants plus sea series participants is greater than the total number of participants. Approximately 5 percent of the participant cohort members were associated with both land and sea series.

TABLE 11-5. Number of Participants* Who Participated in Any Land Series and in Any Sea Series, by Selection Series

Selection Series		Selection Series	Any Land Series	Any Sea Series
GREENHOUSE	Sea	9,528	**781**	9,528
UPSHOT-KNOTHOLE	Land	18,473	18,473	**681**
CASTLE	Sea	15,685	**490**	15,685
REDWING	Sea	12,923	**1,160**	12,923
PLUMBBOB	Land	11,559	11,559	**481**
Total		68,168	32,463	39,298
Participants in both land and sea series			**+2,431**	**+1,162**

NOTE: **Boldface** signifies personnel counted in both "any land" and "any sea" categories.

*No member of the Referent Cohort participated in *any* test series. To maintain comparability between cohorts, referents are assigned the selection series of the matched participant unit.

Table 11-6 shows that for all-cause mortality, land series participants have a slightly, but significantly, lower risk relative to referents (HR = 0.96; 95% CI 0.93–0.99), whereas sea series participants have a slightly higher, also significant, risk relative to sea series referents (HR = 1.03; 95% CI 1.00–1.06). Neither land series nor sea series participants had a significantly higher risk of all-malignancy death (HR = 1.00 and 1.04, respectively). However, land series participants show a statistically significant increase in the hazard ratio for death due to leukemia, 1.49 (1.04–2.13); for sea series participants, the hazard ratio was 0.92 (0.67–1.27), not significantly different from 1.00. Thus, participation in a land series is associated with a significantly higher risk of leukemia death, while participation in a sea series is associated with a significantly increased all-cause death rate.

INVESTIGATING LEUKEMIA RISK BY TIME SINCE FIRST PARTICIPATION AND AGE AT FIRST PARTICIPATION

To explore the increased, but not statistically significant, risk of leukemia observed among participants relative to referents, we looked for patterns consonant with other research findings on the association of radiation and leukemia. We therefore fit a model using time-dependent covariates to estimate the risk of leukemia death in three periods relative to first series participation: less than 5 years, 5 years to less than 15 years, and 15 years or more after participation. We created a model to estimate the risk of leukemia mortality for three ranges of age at first participation: less than 20 years of age, 20 to 25 years, and 25 years and older. Even with this study's very large cohort, there were insufficient early leukemia deaths to yield a definitive picture. Table 11-7 and Table 11-8 (see page 72) show that the relationship between participant status and leukemia mortality does not seem to follow anticipated patterns of latency and age at exposure (Boice, 1996).

TABLE 11-6. Observed Deaths and Hazard Ratio of Participants Relative to Referents, for Land Series and Sea Series Participation

	Land Series[a] (n = 60,227[b])		Sea Series[a] (n = 76,275[b])	
	Observed Deaths	Hazard Ratio[c] (95% CI)	Observed Deaths	Hazard Ratio[c] (95% CI)
All causes	17,586	0.96 (0.93–0.99)	19,676	1.03 (1.00–1.06)
All malignancies	4,719	1.00 (0.95–1.06)	5,373	1.04 (0.98–1.10)
Leukemia minus chronic lymphoid leukemia	135	1.49 (1.04–2.13)	157	0.92 (0.67–1.27)

NOTE: CI = confidence interval.

[a] Attendance at UPSHOT-KNOTHOLE or PLUMBBOB constituted land series participation, regardless of assigned series. Attendance at GREENHOUSE, CASTEL, or REDWING constituted sea series participation, regardless of assigned series. Hence, the number of land participants plus sea participants total more than the overall participant cohort. Members of the referent cohort, however, are assigned to only one series.

[b] Because of missing covariate data, the Proportional Hazards Regression (PHREG) program rejected 22 people having land series participation and 26 having sea series participation.

[c] Participant cohort relative to referent cohort. Proportional hazards model controls for series, service branch, and paygrade by stratification and age at participantion, age squared, and age cubed by covariate adjustment.

TABLE 11-7. Hazard Ratios for Leukemia, Excluding Chronic Lymphoid Leukemia, by Time After First Exposure

Time After First Exposure	Hazard Ratio* (95% CI)
<5 years	0.80 (0.26–2.42)
5 to <15 years	1.09 (0.59–2.02)
≥15 years	1.16 (0.90–1.49)

NOTE: CI = confidence interval.

TABLE 11-8. Hazard Ratios for Leukemia, Excluding Chronic Lymphoid Leukemia, by Age at First Participation

First Participation Age (years)	Hazard Ratio* (95% CI)
<20	1.18 (0.52–2.70)
20 to <25	1.22 (0.81–1.85)
≥25	1.08 (0.79–1.47)

NOTE: CI = confidence interval.

*Participant cohort relative to referent cohort. Proportional hazards model controls for series, service branch, and paygrade by stratification and age, age squared, and age cubed by covariate adjustment.

12

Discussion

In the last chapter of this report of the Five Series Study, we first discuss the principal limitations of the available data. We then discuss our findings (as presented in Chapter 11) in light of the limitations and strengths of these data and the findings that others have reported in studies of atomic veterans.

LIMITATIONS

Fact-of-Death and Cause-of-Death Ascertainment

Death rates for both the participant and the referent cohorts were generally lower than those for the U.S. white male population, resulting in standardized mortality ratios that were nearly all less than 1.0. In part, these low SMRs are due to the "healthy soldier" effect (Seltzer and Jablon, 1974, 1977; see discussion in Appendix C), but underascertainment of fact and cause of death also contributed to lower SMRs.

Among the shortcomings of this analysis are inequalities in the follow-up of participant and referent deaths for which we can assign the cause. For example, we estimated that BIRLS notes roughly 91.8 percent of participant deaths and 90.7 percent of deaths among the referents. In addition, we obtained underlying causes for 95.5 percent of participant deaths but only 92.7 percent of referent deaths (see Chapter 8).

The cumulative effect of these differences is an underascertainment of deaths for which we can assign the cause. For participants, the cumulative ascertainment of deaths with cause is estimated to be 87.7 percent (.918 × .955), and for referents, 84.1 percent (.907 × .927). The net effect of this underascertainment of deaths by cause is to underestimate participant SMRs by roughly 12 percent and referent SMRs by roughly 16 percent. Although we have not corrected the SMRs in our tables for this estimated underascertainment, one could multiply participant SMRs by 1.14 (1 ÷ .877) and referent SMRs by 1.19 (1 ÷ .841) to obtain such an adjustment. Thus, for example, an SMR for participants of 0.75 would be adjusted to 0.86, while the same SMR for referents would yield an adjusted value of 0.89, both values more in keeping with SMR estimates in other military and occupational cohorts.

Further, we point out that such adjustments will not only affect the SMRs, but also the risk estimates we have made. We show the potential effect of underreporting by working through an example, step by step. First, assume that the deaths with unknown cause are distributed in the same fashion as the deaths with cause. Then, taking all cancer mortality as an example (using numbers from Table 11-2), there would have been 231 (i.e., [842 ÷ 18,498] × 5,081) additional deaths observed among participants. The revised SMR is now .78 (i.e., [5,081 + 231] ÷ 6825). For the referent cohort, similar calculations yield a revised SMR of .80, compared to the original value of .74.

Although the calculations above are explicitly made for SMRs, it turns out that (data not shown) the ratio of SMRs is a fairly good empirical approximation to the hazard ratio in this study, probably due in part to the fact that the participant and referent cohorts were frequency matched on age, branch of service, time of service, and paygrade. Thus, although we cannot directly adjust the hazard ratio because we do not have sufficient information, we can use the ratio of the adjusted SMRs to approximate an adjusted hazard ratio. For all cancer deaths, the participants have an adjusted SMR of 0.78, compared to an unadjusted value of 0.74, that is the adjusted SMR is 1.05 times bigger than the unadjusted. For referents, these values are .80 and .74, so that the adjusted SMR is 1.08 times larger. The ratio of the two adjusted SMRs incorporates both of these factors: 0.97 = (.74 × 1.05) ÷ (.74 × 1.08). When rewritten as (.74 ÷ .74) ÷ (1.05 ÷ 1.08), it is clear that the adjusted SMR ratio is the original SMR ratio times an adjustment factor of 0.97 (i.e., 1.05 ÷ 1.08). Within rounding error, this is [1 ÷ .955] divided by [1 ÷ .972], these two quantities being the reciprocals of the percentages of missing causes of death noted above. This further suggests that if we wish to adjust risk ratios (either SMR ratios or hazard ratios) for both missing cause and for unascertained deaths, we should use an adjustment factor of 0.96 (i.e., 1.14 ÷ 1.19; see above). Thus, an estimate for the all cancer hazard ratio adjusted for missing cause of death and for unascertained deaths would be 1.023 × 0.96 = 0.982. Similar calculations yield estimates for adjusted hazard ratios of 1.094 for leukemia minus CLL and 2.232 for thyroid cancer. The effect of this adjustment is always to reduce the size of the original hazard ratios. However, because the same shrinkage factor—0.96—would be applied uniformly to all hazard ratios, we have not displayed adjusted hazard ratios separately.

Stated more generally, the mortality ascertainment was slightly more complete for participants than for referents. This could have contributed to our findings of increased mortality risk among participants. However, we note that all-cause mortality was actually lower among participants than referents. Nonetheless, increased ascertainment of deaths with cause could have contributed to the increased cause-specific risks of death among participants. Although the increased proportion of causes of death among participants is of a much smaller magnitude (roughly 3 percent [4.5% participants, 7.5% referents]) than the increases in leukemia risks we observed (as much as 49% in land series participants), it is possible that ascertainment for certain causes was more differential than the overall difference would suggest.

In this study, mortality ascertainment was hampered by the lack of a nationwide records system that covered the entire study follow-up period. For example, the Health Care Financing Administration of the Department of Health and Human Services tracks Medicare and Medicaid benefit claims, but its database—developed for reasons other than epidemiologic research—does not provide useful information for the years before 1980. Our reliance on data from the National Death Index was limited to deaths since 1979, the year the index was begun. VA records can give information only about those veterans who seek benefits from the VA.

Difficulties remain even when records are available. For example, the coding for cause of death on death certificates is not necessarily uniform across geographic regions or time periods, or across the various groups of personnel responsible for choosing which cause, among the overlapping possibilities, to formalize on a death certificate.

Statistical Power

Veteran concern about radiogenic cancer was a major impetus for this research. That leukemia, the cancer that is most consistently linked with radiation, is fairly rare is fortunate overall but presents an obstacle to a study of this kind. Only a study cohort four times the size of the one available would have been likely to identify the observed leukemia risk as statistically significant. The sample size presently available does not provide sufficient power to achieve statistical significance for risks of the magnitudes we observed.

Other Possible Confounding Factors

Military Service Characteristics

Within the military, most personnel serve for a discrete time period and then proceed into the civilian arena of work and life. Others choose a military career and remain in the service. The two sets of personnel may have different characteristics. Career military personnel, similar to many but not all occupational groups, must maintain reasonably good health to remain in the military, making them a healthy cohort. However, if one's military occupation involves, for ex ample, radiation exposure, longer service could involve higher cumulative doses. Had individual-level data been available on length of service and job categories (as proxies for potential hazardous exposures), we might have been able to identify differences between the participant and referent cohorts, if any, that may have confounded associations between participation and mortality.

Other Lifetime Radiation Exposure

We have no information on other lifetime radiation exposure to members of either cohort either before or after the time period of the atomic tests. Sources of dose include background radiation, medical procedures (diagnostic and therapeutic), and occupational practices (civilian and military). Only if additional exposures were substantially unequal in the two cohorts could they create a bias.

Contributing and Associated Causes of Death

We did not analyze data on associated causes of death (i.e., those noted on the death certificate in addition to the underlying cause). In the case of leukemia minus chronic lymphoid leukemia, this was not an important shortcoming, since only two leukemia minus CLL deaths were listed as associated and not underlying causes of death. There may have been other mortality outcomes, however, for which an analysis of associated causes would be more fruitful.

Inadequate Dosimetry

Although the oversight committee concluded that the dose data in their current form were unsuitable for epidemiologic analysis (IOM, 1995), it also concluded that carefully done custom dose reconstructions performed anew for selected participants using consistent methods could provide usable dose data. Such custom dose reconstructions, however, would be prohibitively expensive to carry out for the entire cohort of participants. A more efficient way to make use of custom dose data would be to undertake a further study using a nested case-control design (Rothman and Greenland, 1998). Briefly, leukemia deaths among participants could be selected for study, along with a randomly sampled control group (also of participants). Radiation dose would be estimated for everyone in the study using custom dose reconstructions, and the pattern of radiation dose among the leukemia deaths could be contrasted to the pattern among the selected participant controls. In particular, dose–response analyses could be undertaken using such a study design.

Other research options include identifying incident cases of cancers. Such information would assist in understanding the association of radiation with non-fatal cancers. The absence of a national cancer registry would hamper any study of cancer incidence or prevalence. Alternative sources of information could include geographically specific or disease-specific registries, health insurance claim data, and treatment data sources.

DISCUSSION

The data presented in Chapter 11, based on more than 5 million person-years of mortality follow-up, represent one of the largest cohort studies of military veterans ever conducted. Overall, no statistically significant differences in all-cause, all-cancer, or leukemia[*] mortality between participants and referents are evident, although the participant risk of leukemia death is 14 percent higher than the referent risk.

Across broad categories of noncancer deaths, participants and referents had the same mortality risk, except for death due to external causes, for which participants had a significantly higher risk (HR = 1.08; 95% C.I. 1.02–1.16; see Table 11-2). Neither information about the nuclear tests nor current understanding of radiobiology helps us to explain this observed higher risk. Similar estimates of excess mortality due to external causes, however, have been found in the study of British nuclear test participants (relative risk 1.06 for the initial follow-up through 1983 and 1.03 for 1984 through 1990; Darby et al., 1993b), New Zealand nuclear test participants (1.10; Pearce et al., 1997), as well as other military populations in Vietnam and the Persian Gulf (Kang and Bullman, 1996; Thomas et al., 1991; USDHHS, 1987; Watanabe and Kang, 1995). Conversely, participants in Operation CROSSROADS had a lower risk for deaths due to accidents relative to their referent group (HR = 0.98) (Johnson et al., 1996).

In the following section of the report, we include discussion of the cancer findings that (1) relate to leukemia, a predetermined analytic endpoint; (2) are of interest because they relate to organs that are known to respond to radiation or have been identified in other studies of atomic test participants—thyroid and lung cancers; or (3) are statistically significant—nasal and prostate cancers.

Leukemia

For all leukemias and leukemia minus CLL we found increased, not statistically significant, hazard ratios. Other studies of atomic veterans provide mixed evidence for radiogenic leukemia. In our earlier mortality study of Operation CROSSROADS participation (Johnson et al., 1996), we reported a not statistically significant increase in leukemia deaths among participants relative to referents. However, Darby and colleagues (1993a,b) found a statistically significant

[*]Based on current expert understanding of radiogenicity, we define *leukemia* throughout this chapter as ICD-9 codes 204 to 208 *excluding 204.1, chronic lymphoid leukemia.* Other use of the term leukemia is noted in the text.

increase in leukemia deaths (RR = 1.75; 90% CI 1.01–3.06) among British participants in nuclear tests in Australia and the Pacific. The rate was higher (RR = 3.45; 90% CI 1.50–8.38) when limited to the earlier years of follow-up (Darby et al., 1988a,b). Similarly, Pearce and colleagues (1996, 1997) found a statistically significant increase in leukemia deaths (RR = 5.59; 90% CI 1.04–41.7) among New Zealand test participants.

Arguing against a radiogenic cause for the leukemia excess among American atomic test series veterans is the finding from Watanabe and colleagues (1995) that highly exposed (>1,000 mrem) participants had no significant excess leukemia mortality. However, Watanabe's study used only sea series nuclear test participants and dose measures that the IOM advisory committee found to be inappropriate for epidemiologic analysis. We too found no increased risk of leukemia among sea series participants (HR = 0.92; 95% CI 0.67–1.27).

We found that land series participants, relative to land series referents, were at a statistically significant increased estimated risk of death due to leukemia (HR = 1.49; 95% CI 1.04–2.13). For all causes of death, sea series participation was associated with a statistically significant lower mortality risk; land series participants and referents were essentially equal. However, we cannot rule out the possibility that the excess leukemia in land participants is due to chance.

Although the data are far from definitive, our findings are broadly consistent with a radiogenic basis for the excess leukemia deaths observed. The relative risks for leukemia deaths were highest for two acute leukemia subtypes— lymphoid leukemia excluding chronic lymphoid leukemia and myeloid leukemia excluding chronic myeloid leukemia (Table 11-4). However, neither the pattern of leukemia deaths by follow-up period nor the pattern by age at test series participation serves to strengthen the evidence of a radiogenic relationship, although we had limited statistical power to analyze such patterns. We also made only preliminary investigations of leukemia minus CLL risk patterns by branch, paygrade, and participation status (see Appendix E).

Thyroid Cancer

Although thyroid cancer is one of the four cancers (leukemia, lung, and breast cancers are the other three) with strong evidence for radiation risk (Boice, 1996), the evidence relates almost entirely to childhood exposure. In fact, available evidence suggests that the adult thyroid gland is relatively insensitive to induction from radiation exposure (Hall et al., 1996; IOM, 1999; Thompson et al., 1994).

Although there were only 18 thyroid cancer deaths observed, we looked at the hazard of thyroid cancer deaths by age at first nuclear test participation. The results were not consistent with what we expected based on the literature: the hazard ratio (of participants relative to referents) was higher for those age 22 and older than for those less than age 22 at the time of participation.

Explanations of the apparent increased rate of thyroid cancer deaths among participants—aside from a radiation effect—include increased surveillance among participants, chance, and differential ascertainment of causes of death for the participant and referent deaths. In considering the possibility of increased detection of thyroid cancers among participants, we note the possible incentive for participants to seek screening tests more aggressively out of both a concern about prior radiation exposure and the knowledge that thyroid cancer is compensable under VA regulations. More cases identified could result in more diagnoses noted on the death certificate. Because thyroid cancer has a relatively low (10 percent) fatality rate, a few additional found cases *could* influence the study findings.

Neither the Darby nor Pearce team found an increased risk of death due to thyroid cancer; Watanabe et al. did not present data on this site. However, Johnson and colleagues reported an HR of 3.48 for thyroid cancer mortality among Operation CROSSROADS participants, not statistically significant, but still the highest relative risk reported.

Lung Cancer

Although evidence for the radiogenicity of lung cancer is strong (Boice, 1996), the well-documented association between smoking and lung cancer—and our lack of data on smoking—make an interpretation of any association problematic. Indeed, there is a particular interest in the interaction of the effects of tobacco smoke and radiation (Mettler and Upton, 1995).

We found no evidence of an increased risk among participants of death due to lung cancer (HR 0.99; 95% CI 0.93–1.06). This is consistent with the nonsignificant findings of all the other follow-up studies of nuclear weapons test participants: Darby and colleagues (1993a,b), 0.85 (90% CI 0.73–0.99); Pearce and colleagues (Pearce, 1996; Pearce et al., 1997), 0.94 (90% CI 0.45–1.84); Watanabe and colleagues (1995), 1.16 (95% CI 0.66–2.05) in the high-exposure group and 1.07 (95% CI 0.83–1.38) overall; and Johnson and colleagues (1996), 1.05 (95% CI 0.96–1.14).

Nasal Cancer

We found an excess risk of mortality attributed to nasal cancer in this study, but other studies have not reported similar results. For example, no increase in nasal and pharyngeal cancer has been seen in Japanese atomic bomb survivors (Schull, 1995). In their textbook on medical effects of ionizing radiation, Mettler and Upton (1995) listed the nasal sinuses as having low susceptibility to radiation-induced cancers compared to other sites listed as high or moderate. Johnson et al. (1996) did not look specifically at nasal cancers in their study of mortality associated with participation in the CROSSROADS nuclear test series. However, going back to that dataset, we find a hazard ratio of 6.70 (95% CI 0.82– 54.49).

Prostate Cancer

Prostate cancer is not generally thought to be caused by radiation (Mettler and Upton, 1995), and no increase in prostate cancer has been seen among Japanese atomic bomb survivors (Schull, 1995). Although data from the ankylosing spondylitis cohort (Darby et al., 1987) pointed to an early excess of prostate cancer, the authors noted that prostate cancer and ankylosing spondylitis can be confused, due to the presence of back pain from prostate cancer metastases to the spine. In addition, there have been a number of studies of occupational cohorts, with varying results (see Mettler and Upton, 1995; National Research Council, 1990).

Studies of nuclear weapons test participants have also yielded varying resuits. Darby and colleagues (1993a,b) found a relative risk of 0.93 (90% CI 0.62–1.41); Pearce and colleagues (Pearce, 1996; Pearce et al., 1997), 0.35 (90% CI 0.02–2.08); Watanabe and colleagues (1995), 1.46 (95% CI 0.34–6.31) in the high-exposure group and 1.41 (95% CI 0.71–2.80) overall; and Johnson and colleagues (1996), 0.77 (95% CI 0.61–0.97). Thus, except for Johnson, who found a statistically significant deficit in prostate mortality risk, and the present study, which found a statistically significant excess risk (HR 1.20; 95% CI 1.03– 1.40), all other studies of nuclear weapons test participants have found no statistically significant excess or deficit in risk.

Given the generally negative prostate findings reported in other studies, we urge caution in the interpretation of our findings. Moreover, a complicating factor in the study of prostate cancer is the large proportion of undiagnosed prostate cancers (Mettler and Upton, 1995), which could have affected our resuits. Specifically, participant concerns about the possibility of cancer being caused by their participation may have led to more intensive follow-up, with a concomitant increase in prostate cancer discovered, and subsequently, in reported deaths due to prostate cancer.

CONCLUDING COMMENTS

Having described the difficulties faced in carrying out this study—most of which are shared by other studies involving insufficiently recorded exposure and endpoint information, we here recapitulate some of its general advantages. First, in contrast to the earlier study by the Medical Follow-up Agency (Robinette et al., 1985), we now have more confidence that the five series participants have been properly identified (see Appendix D). The present study also makes use of a military referent cohort, rather than relying solely on standardized mortality ratios based on U.S. population controls. There is also a longer mortality follow-up period. In comparison to other studies of nuclear test participants, the Five Series Study's inclusion of more than 68,000 participants surpasses in size any previous research.

It is unlikely that another cohort study of this type and magnitude would provide more precise answers than this, because any atomic veteran study of this kind would face the same methodologic problems—namely, inadequate exposure data and imperfect mortality ascertainment—that we encountered in this Five Series Study. Other research strategies, using better-defined dosimetry data, might be those that focus on specific diseases and more detailed individual-level exposure information.

The size, length of follow-up, and persistence of data collection efforts involved in this Five Series Study have helped to assure us that the findings we report are valid. The weak associations observed and the varied consistency with other studies, however, make interpreting these findings difficult.

We can state that the participant group *as a whole* did not experience widespread early death. Even for leukemia, for example, there were an estimated 25 excess deaths in the participant cohort. That might be a comfort to those veterans who are not sick and to their families. The report findings do not rule out, however, possible increased risk among distinct subgroups of test participants.

References

Allison PD. *Survival Analysis Using the SAS System: A Practical Guide*. Cary, N.C. : SAS Institute Inc. , 1995 .

AMA (American Medical Association). *Encyclopedia of Medicine*. C Clayman (ed.). New York : Random House , 1989 .

Berkhouse L , Davis SE , Gladeck FR , Hallowell JH , Jones CB , Martin EJ , McMullan FW , Osborne MJ. *Operation Greenhouse—1951*. DNA-6034F . Washington, D.C. : Defense Nuclear Agency , 1983 .

Boice, JD Jr. Risk Estimates for Radiation Exposures . Pp. 237–268 in WR Hendee and FM Edwards (eds.) *Health Effects of Exposure to Low-Level Ionizing Radiation* . Philadelphia : Institute of Physics Publishing , 1996 .

Boice JD Jr. , Engholm G , Kleinerman RA , et al. Radiation dose and second cancer risk in patients treated for cancer of the cervix . *Radiation Research* 116 : 3–55 , 1988 .

Boice JD Jr. , Land CE , Preston DL. Ionizing Radiation . Pp. 319–354 in D Schottenfeld and JF Fraumeni, Jr. (eds.) *Cancer Epidemiology and Prevention* , 2nd edition . New York : Oxford University Press , 1996 .

Boice JD Jr. , Monson RR , Rosenstein M. Cancer mortality in women after repeated fluoroscopic examinations of the chest . *Journal of the National Cancer Institute* 66 : 863–867 , 1981 .

Boice JD Jr. , Rosenstein M , Trout DE. Estimation of breast cancer doses and breast cancer risk associated with repeated fluoroscopic chest examinations of women with tuberculosis . *Radiation Research* 73 : 373–390 , 1978 .

Boyle CA , Decoufle P. National sources of vital status information: Extent of coverage and possible selectivity in reporting . *American Journal of Epidemiology* 132 : 1196–1197 , 1990 .

Bruce-Henderson S , Gladeck F , Hallowell J , Martin E , McMullan F , Miller R , Rogers W , Rowland R , Shelton C. *Operation Redwing: 1956*. DNA 6037F . Washington, D.C. : Defense Nuclear Agency , 1982 .

Caldwell GG , Kelley D , Heath CW Jr. Leukemia among participants in military maneuvers at a nuclear bomb test: A preliminary report . *Journal of the American Medical Association* 244 (14) : 1575–1578 , 1980 .

Caldwell GG , Kelley D , Zack M , Falk H , Heath, CW Jr. Mortality and cancer frequency among military nuclear test (SMOKY) participants, 1957 through 1979 . *Journal of the American Medical Association* 250(5) : 620–624 , 1983 .

CFR (Code of Federal Regulations). "Standards for Protection Against Radiation: Final Rule." Title 10, Pt. 20 , 1991 .

CFR. "Claims Under the Radiation Exposure Compensation Act." Title 28, Pt 79.41 , 1998a .

CFR. "Diseases Subject to Presumptive Service Connection." Title 38, Pt. 3.309 , 1998b .

Cox DR. Regression models and lifetables [with discussion] . *Journal of the Royal Statistical Society* 34B : 187–220 , 1972 .

Darby SC , Doll R , Gill SK , Smith PG. Long term mortality after a single treatment course with x-rays in patients treated for ankylosing spondylitis . *British Journal of Cancer* 55(2) : 179–190 , 1987 .

Darby SC , Kendall GM , Fell TP , Doll R , Goodill AA , Conquest AH , Jackson DA , Haylock RGE. *Mortality and Cancer Incidence 1952–1990 in UK Participants in the UK Atmospheric Nuclear Weapon Tests and Experimental Programmes.* Report No. NRPB-R266 . Oxon, United Kingdom : National Radiological Protection Board , 1993a .

Darby SC , Kendall GM , Fell TP , Doll R , Goodill AA , Conquest AH , Jackson DA , Haylock RGE. Further follow up of mortality and incidence of cancer in men from the United Kingdom who participated in the United Kingdom's atmospheric nuclear weapon tests and experimental programmes . *British Medical Journal* 307 : 1530–1535 , 1993b .

Darby SC , Kendall GM , Fell TP , O'Hagan JA , Muirhead CR , Ennis JR , Ball AM , Dennis JA , Doll R. *Mortality and Cancer Incidence in UK Participants in UK Atmospheric Nuclear Weapon Tests and Experimental Programmes.* Report No. NPRB-R214 . Oxon, United Kingdom : National Radiological Protection Board , 1988a .

Darby SC , Kendall GM , Fell TP , O'Hagan JA , Muirhead CR , Ennis JR , Ball AM , Dennis JA , Doll R. A summary of mortality and incidence of cancer in men from the United Kingdom who participated in the United Kingdom's atmospheric nuclear weapon tests and experimental programmes . *British Medical Journal* 296 : 332–338 , 1988b .

DNA (Defense Nuclear Agency). Fact Sheet: Greenhouse Fact Sheet . Washington, D.C. : Defense Nuclear Agency, Public Affairs Office , 1981 (unpublished) .

DNA. Fact Sheet: Operation Upshot-Knothole . Washington, D.C. : Defense Nuclear Agency, Public Affairs Office , 1982 (unpublished) .

DSWA (Defense Special Weapons Agency). Letter dated 28 February 1997, with data tapes attached, from DM Schaeffer, NTPR Program Manager, Electronics and Systems Directorate, Defense Special Weapons Agency to JC Johnson, Medical Follow-up Agency .

DTRA (Defense Threat Reduction Agency). Radiation Exposure in U.S. Atmospheric Nuclear Weapons Testing, Nuclear Test Personnel Review Program . [www document]: http://www.dtra.mil/news/facts/ntprpre.html , 1999 .

Fisher SB , Weber L , Goldberg J , Davis F. Mortality ascertainment in the veteran population: Alternatives to the National Death Index . *American Journal of Epidemiology* 141 : 242–250 , 1995 .

GAO (General Accounting Office). *Mortality Study of Atmospheric Nuclear Test Participants Is Flawed.* Report to the Chairman, Committee on Veterans' Affairs, U.S. Senate Report No. GAO/RCED-92-182 . Washington, D.C. : U.S. General Accounting Office , August 1992 .

Gelband H. *A Discussion of Questions About the 1985 NAS Report* "Mortality of Nuclear Weapons Test Participants." Washington, D.C. : Office of Technology Assessment , August 1992 .

Gladeck F , Johnson A. *For the Record: A History of the Nuclear Test Personnel Review Program, 1978–1993.* DNA-6041F . Washington, D.C. : Defense Nuclear Agency , 1996 .

Hall P , Mattson A , and Boice JD Jr. Thyroid cancer diagnostic administration of iodine-131 . *Radiation Research* 145 : 86–92 , 1996 .

Harris P , Lowery C , Nelson A , Obermiller S , Ozeroff W , Weary S. *Plumbbob Series, 1957.* Washington, D.C. : Defense Nuclear Agency , 1981 .

ICRP (International Commission on Radiological Protection). Nonstochastic effects of ionizing radiation . ICRP Publication 41 . *Annals of the ICRP* 14(3) , 1984 .

ICRP. 1990 recommendations of the International Commission on Radiological Protection . ICRP Publication 60 . *Annals of the ICRP* 21(1–3) , 1991 .

IOM (Institute of Medicine). *A Review of the Dosimetry Data Available in the Nuclear Test Personnel Review (NTPR) Program.* An Interim Letter Report of the Committee to Study the Mortality of Military Personnel Present at Atmospheric Tests of Nuclear Weapons to the Defense Nuclear Agency . Washington, D.C. : Institute of Medicine , 1995 .

IOM. *Exposure of the American People to Iodine-131 from Nevada Nuclear-Bomb Tests: Review of the National Cancer Institute Report and Public Health Implications.* Washington, D.C. : National Academy Press , 1999 .

JAYCOR. 5 Series Cohort Unit Selection Methodology Report for the National Academy of Sciences . Provided by DM Schaeffer, Defense Nuclear Agency , June 1995 (unpublished document) .

JAYCOR. Participant Identification Methodology Report for the National Academy of Sciences . Provided by DM Schaeffer, Defense Nuclear Agency , June 1997 (unpublished document) .

Johnson AA , Goetz JL , McRaney WK. *For the Record: A History of the Nuclear Test Personnel Review Program, 1978–1986.* DNA-6041F . Washington, D.C. : Defense Nuclear Agency , 1986 .

Johnson JC , Thaul S , Page WF , Crawford H. *Mortality of Veteran Participants in the CROSSROADS Nuclear Test.* Washington, D.C. : National Academy Press , 1996 .

Kang HK , Bullman TA. Mortality among U.S. veterans of the Persian Gulf War . *New England Journal of Medicine* 335 : 1498–1504 , 1996 .

Korn EL , Graubard BI , Midthune D. Time-to-event analysis of longitudinal follow-up of a survey: Choice of the time scale . *American Journal of Epidemiology* 145(1) : 72–80 , 1997 .

Land CE. Studies of cancer and radiation dose among atomic bomb survivors: The example of breast cancer . *Journal of the American Medical Association* , 1995 .

Last JM. *A Dictionary of Epidemiology* , 3rd edition . New York : Oxford University Press , 1995 .

Mabuchi K , Soda M , Ron E , Tokunaga M , Ochikubo S , Sugimoto S , Ikeda T , Terasaki M , Preston DL , Thompson DE. Cancer incidence in atomic bomb survivors. Part I: Use of the tumor registries in Hiroshima and Nagasaki for incidence studies . *Radiation Research* . 137(Suppl.) : S1–S16 , 1994 .

Marsh GM , Youk AO , Stone RA , Sefcik S , Alcorn C. OCMAP-PLUS: A program for the comprehensive analysis of occupational cohort data . *Journal of Occupational and Environmental Medicine* 40 : 351–362 , 1998 .

Martin E , Rowland R. *Castle Series, 1954*. DNA 6035 F . Washington, D.C. : Defense Nuclear Agency , 1982 .

Mettler FA , Upton AC. *Medical Effects of Ionizing Radiation* , 2nd ed. Philadelphia : W.B. Saunders , 1995 .

Nagataki S , Shibata Y , Inoue S , Yokoyama N , Izumi M , Shimaoka K. Thyroid diseases among atomic bomb survivors in Nagasaki . *Journal of the American Medical Association* 272 (5) : 364–370 , 1994 .

NCRP (National Council on Radiation Protection and Measurements). *Ionizing Radiation Exposure of the Population of the United States*. NCRP Report. No. 93 . Bethesda, Md. : National Council on Radiation Protection and Measurements , 1987 .

National Research Council. Committee on the Biological Effects of Ionizing Radiation (BEIR V). *Health Effects of Exposure to Low Levels of Ionizing Radiation*. Washington, D.C. : National Academy Press , 1990 .

Page WF. VA mortality reporting for World War II Army veterans [letter] . *American Journal of Public Health* 82(1) : 124–125 , 1992 .

Page WF. *Evaluation of Vietnam Veteran Mortality Ascertainment by Department of Veterans Affairs Files*, Final report to the Veterans Administration under contract V101(93)P-1316 . Washington, D.C. , March 1993 (unpublished manuscript) .

Page WF , Braun MM , Caporaso NE. Ascertainment of mortality in the U.S. veteran population: World War II veteran twins . *Military Medicine* 160(7) : 351–355 , 1995 .

Page WF , Mahan CM , Kang HK. Vital status ascertainment through the files of the Department of Veterans Affairs and the Social Security Administration . *Annals of Epidemiology* 6(2) : 102–109 , 1996 .

Pearce N. *Mortality and Cancer Incidence in New Zealand Participants in United Kingdom Nuclear Weapons Tests in the Pacific: Supplementary Report*. Wellington, New Zealand : Wellington School of Medicine , 1996 .

Pearce N , Winkelmann R , Kennedy J , Lewis S , Purdie G , Slater T , Prior I , Fraser J. Further follow-up of New Zealand participants in United Kingdom atmospheric nuclear weapons tests in the Pacific . *Cancer Causes and Control* 8 : 139–145 , 1997 .

Pierce DA , Shimizu Y , Preston DL , Vaeth M , Mabuchi K. Studies of the mortality of A-bomb survivors. Report 12, Part I. Cancer: 1950–1990 . *Radiation Research* 146 : 1–27 , 1996 .

Ponton J , Massie J , Maag C , Shepanel R , Rohrer S. *Operation Upshot-Knothole, 1953*. Washington, D.C. : Defense Nuclear Agency , 1982 .

Preston DL , Kusumi S , Tomonaga M , Izumi S , Ron E , Kuramoto A , Kamada N , Dohy H , Matsui T , Nonaka H , Thompson DE , Soda M , Mabuchi K. Cancer incidence inatomic bomb survivors. Part III: Leukemia, lymphoma and multiple myeloma, 1950–1987 . *Radiation Research* 137(Suppl.) : S68–S97 , 1994 .

Robinette CD , Jablon S , Preston TL. *Mortality of Nuclear Weapons Test Participants*. Washington, D.C. : National Research Council , 1985 .

Ron E. Ionizing radiation and cancer risk: Evidence from epidemiology . *Radiation Research* 150 (Suppl.) : S30–S41 , 1998 .

Ron E , Preston DL , Mabuchi K , Thompson DE , Soda M. Cancer incidence in atomic bomb survivors. Part IV: Comparison of cancer incidence and mortality . *Radiation Research* 137 (Suppl.) : S98–S112 , 1994 .

Rothman KJ and Greenland S. *Modern Epidemiology*. 2nd edition . Philadelphia : Lippincott-Raven , 1998 .

SAS Institute, Inc. *SAS/STAT Software: Changes and Enhancements Through Release 6.11*. Cary, N.C. : SAS Institute, Inc. , 1996 .

Schull WJ. *Effects of Atomic Radiation: A Half-Century of Studies from Hiroshima and Nagasaki.* New York : Wiley-Liss , 1995 .

Seltzer CC , Jablon S. Effects of selection on mortality . *American Journal of Epidemiology* 100 : 367–372 , 1974 .

Seltzer CC , Jablon S. Army rank and subsequent mortality by cause: 23-year follow-up . *American Journal of Epidemiology* 105 : 559–566 , 1977 .

Sherman GJ , Howe GR , Miller AB , Rosenstein M. Organ dose per unit exposure resulting from fluoroscopy for artificial pneumothorax . *Health Physics* 35 : 259–269 , 1978 .

Shore RE , Hildreth N , Woodward E , Dvoretsky P , Hempelmann L , Pasternack B. Breast cancer among women given x-ray therapy for acute postpartum mastitis . *Journal of the National Cancer Institute* 77(3) : 689–696 , 1986 .

Singleton RA , Straits BC , Straits MM. *Approaches to Social Research.* 2nd edition . New York : Oxford University Press , 1993 .

Thomas, TL , Kang HK , Dalager NA. Mortality among women Vietnam veterans, 1973–1987 . *American Journal of Epidemiology* 134 : 973–980 , 1991 .

Thompson DE , Mabuchi K , Ron E , Soda M , Tokunaga M , Ochobuko S , Sugimoto S , Ikeda T , Terasaki M , Izumi S , et al. Cancer incidence in atomic bomb survivors. Part II: Solid tumors . *Radiation Research* 137(Suppl.) : S17–S67 , 1994 .

UNSCEAR (United Nations Scientific Committee on the Effects of Atomic Radiation). *Sources and Effects of Ionizing Radiation.* UNSCEAR 1994 Report to the General Assembly with Scientific Annexes . New York : United Nations , 1994 .

USDHHS (U.S. Department of Health and Human Services). Postservice mortality among Vietnam veterans (The Centers for Disease Control Vietnam Experience Study) . *Journal of the American Medical Association* 257(6) : 790–795 , 1987 .

USDHHS. The *International Classification of Diseases, Ninth Revision, Clinical Modification*, 4th edition . DHHS Publication No. (PHS) 91-1260) , 1991 .

Watanabe KK , Kang HK. Military service in Vietnam and the risk of death from trauma and selected cancers . *Annals of Epidemiology* 5 : 407–412 , 1995 .

Watanabe KK , Kang HK , Dalager NA. Cancer mortality risk among military participants of a 1958 atmospheric nuclear weapons test . *American Journal of Public Health* 85 : 523 , 1995 .

APPENDIX A

A Review of the Dosimetry Data Available in the Nuclear Test Personnel Review Program

This appendix contains a reprint of *A Review of the Dosimetry Data Available in the Nuclear Test Personnel Review Program: An Interim Letter Report of the Committee to Study the Mortality of Military Personnel Present at Atmos pheric Tests of Nuclear Weapons to the Defense Nuclear Agency,* which was delivered to the agency on 15 May 1995.

Committee with broad expertise in biostatistics, uncertainty analysis, environmental dosimetry, dose assessment, and health physics. The Five-Series Committee has carefully scrutinized the information presented to it by the Working Group and has prepared this interim letter report to document its findings and conclusions.

The objective of the Working Group was to determine whether doses that have been assigned to the Atomic Veterans and entered into the database of the NTPR program can be used as a basis for dose-response analysis in the Five-Series Study. The Working Group reviewed dose-related fields contained in the NTPR database and the methods used to estimate doses. The review considered four criteria that, ideally, should be applied when generating dose data for an epidemiologic study: (1) consistency in the technical approach, (2) nondifferential methods of dose assignment, (3) quality assurance, and (4) application of uncertainty analysis. The Working Group held discussions with NTPR staff who are involved in the dosimetry and reviewed printouts of the NTPR database, as well as files of specific veterans for whom individualized doses have been determined.

The Working Group concluded that there has been a lack of consistency over time in NTPR dose estimation methods and, in particular, in the methods of assigning "high-sided" doses, that is, doses in which uncertainties are resolved in favor of assigning higher doses rather than lower doses. In some cases, because of the existing compensation program, procedures for assigning doses have been different for those who did and did not file a claim for a radiogenic cancer. Neither the dose assignment methods nor the database itself are thoroughly documented. In addition, uncertainties have not been estimated in a consistent manner and do not incorporate all potential sources of variability inherent in the dosimetry.

The Working Group, therefore, concludes that the NTPR dose data are not suitable for dose-response analysis. This conclusion is based on the fact that the NTPR dose data were based on incomplete records, were developed primarily for the purpose of ensuring appropriate follow-up for participating veterans and do not meet the particular standards needed for use in epidemiologic research. The Working Group believes, based on its review, that comprehensive dose reconstructions may be feasible for a limited subset of veterans who participated in the above ground nuclear test program. If doses on this population are required for epidemiologic purposes, they should be recalculated according to the fundamental principles described in this report.

OBJECTIVES OF THE DOSIMETRY WORKING GROUP

The Medical Follow-up Agency (MFUA) of the IOM is undertaking a 5-year study to evaluate the mortality experience of military personnel, the atomic veterans, who participated in at least one of Five-Series of atmospheric nuclear weapons tests during the period 1951– 1957. The principal purpose of the study is to ascertain whether mortality from leukemias, other cancers, or any other diseases has occurred at a higher rate among participants in atmospheric nuclear weapon tests compared with a similar group of veterans who were not participants. For additional background on the study and the IOM committee overseeing it, see Appendix A.

As initially planned, the study would utilize participant identification and radiation exposure data provided by the Defense Nuclear Agency (DNA) of the Department of Defense (DoD). In designing the study protocol, the committee recommended that the dosimetry assignments for the Five-Series personnel be evaluated for the purpose of this epidemiologic study. To conduct this review, the committee constituted a working group with expertise in dose reconstruction, environmental transport of radionuclides, uncertainty analysis, measurement and dosimetry techniques, general health physics, and statistics. The Dosimetry Working Group roster is provided as Appendix B.

The Working Group recognizes that dosimetry data could yield valuable insights into a dose-response relationship for an epidemiologic analysis, if they were derived from specific information that characterizes the veteran's duties at the time of his participation in the weapons tests and if they were estimated in a consistent and well-documented manner. The Working Group also understands that the NTPR database was developed primarily for the purposes of responding to veterans' inquiries about radiation exposures and as a basis for providing appropriate follow-up and settling claims for compensation in accordance with federal regulations. Furthermore, it is apparent that the NTPR database has evolved over a period of time (Appendix C) that has seen improvements in the state of the art of dosimetric methods, advances in uncertainty analysis, and further discovery and review of historical records.

The objective of the Working Group, therefore, was to evaluate NTPR dosimetry with an eye toward its applicability in an epidemiologic study. The Working Group did so by reviewing relevant documentation; tracing the origin of several individual dose assignments; and comparing the methods used with those generally acceptable for epidemiologic analysis.

PREVIOUS NRC REPORTS ON NTPR DOSIMETRY

The National Research Council (NRC) previously published two reports on dosimetry related to exposures of participants in atmospheric nuclear weapon tests. The first report, "Review of the Methods Used to Assign Radiation Doses to Service Personnel at Nuclear Weapons Tests," (NRC, 1985a) advised the DNA on whether the methods used by NTPR to assign doses of radiation are comprehensive and scientifically sound, and recommended improvements. The second report, "Film Badge Dosimetry in Atmospheric Nuclear Tests," (NRC, 1989) was an in-depth evaluation of film badge dosimetry practices used during the weapons testing period, recording and record-keeping of dosimetric data, and overall uncertainties associated with the film badge readings. Neither of these reports, however, judged the feasibility of using NTPR dose data as the basis for epidemiologic analysis.

EVALUATION CRITERIA EMPLOYED BY THE WORKING GROUP

In its review, the Working Group considered four criteria that, ideally, should be met if dose estimates are to be useful in an epidemiologic study. Criteria used included (1) consistency in the technical approach, (2) nondifferential methods of dose assignment, (3) quality assurance, and (4) uncertainty analysis. A brief description of these criteria follows.

Consistency in the Technical Approach

Ideally, consistent methods should be applied to assigning doses to all subjects contained in the database. Algorithms used to estimate doses should be uniform from one subject to the next. Assumptions made to permit calculations of dose in cases in which no physical dosimetry data are available should be applied uniformly among the study population. If there is a tendency to bias doses in either direction, the bias applied should also be incorporated into each dose assignment. This consistency is crucial to successful merging of *individual* dosimetry with *individual* effects data for use in an epidemiologic study.

Nondifferential Methods of Dose Assignment

Dose assignment methods should not differ for individuals who were made known to NTPR because they or their surrogate filed a claim for compensation versus those who did not. If veterans who developed leukemia and filed a claim, for example, were assigned doses by methods that systematically differed from those used to assign doses to veterans who have never filed a claim, then this could produce serious bias in evaluating the dose-response relationship between radiation exposure and leukemia mortality.

Quality Assurance

Ideally, there should be comprehensive documentation of both the methods used to determine doses and the individual dose assignments. Each dose should be traceable and capable of being recalculated through documentation. It is important to document methods as actually applied, such as the algorithms applied (for dosimetry and uncertainty), parameters used (and associated distributions), assumptions regarding scenarios of exposure, and default values included when data are not available, as well as verification of data entry. A careful audit trail would allow any corrections that had been made over time to the person's assigned dose to be retraced. Mathematical models estimating doses should also be tested to compare predicted results to measured values.

Uncertainty Analysis

Significant advances have been made over the past decade in the analysis of uncertainty for environmental dose analysis. Current state-of-the-art environmental dosimetry requires quantitatively deriving best dose estimates coupled with associated uncertainties. Uncertainties should account for all possible sources of bias, including modeling bias, parameter bias, and parameter variability. To be most useful for the Five-Series Study, unbiased best estimates of dose should be bounded by a range that indicates the degree of subjective confidence.

REVIEW PROCESS

The Working Group met twice, once on 12–13 April 1994 and once on 16–17 May 1994. Both meetings were held in Washington, D.C. Prior to its first meeting, the Working Group was provided with background material on the NTPR program (Appendix D). On 12 April, the Working Group received briefings by Mr. D. M. Schaeffer of DNA on the NTPR database and Dr. W. J. Klemm of Science Applications International Corporation (SAIC) on dose assessment methods. The Working Group devoted considerable time to understanding the methods used in assigning doses and building and maintaining the NTPR database. On 13 April, the Working Group made site visits to JAYCOR and SAIC to review pertinent records. This review included documentation of methodologies, dose assignment policies, records from the NTPR database, and files of individual participants.

At its second meeting, the Working Group reviewed additional information and drafted its report for the Five Series Committee. Upon receiving the report, the full committee carefully scrutinized the information presented to it by the Working Group and prepared this interim letter report to document its findings and conclusions.

OBSERVATIONS

The NTPR Database

The NTPR database contains the following categories of information:

- personal identification and information related to claims, cause of death, etc.;
- records of correspondence sent by the DNA;
- duty assignments and intervals of participation for specific test series;
- dose assignments obtained from dosimetry records;
- dose assignments derived by reconstruction; and,
- total doses by test series and summed across all series combined.

Individual fields contain codes that identify results, explanations, sources of information, and so on (Appendix E).

The dose estimates entered into the database may be derived from film badges, dose reconstructions, a combination of the two, or from other sources. The ideal dose estimates are those based on undamaged badges actually worn by the individual during that person's entire time of participation in atmospheric tests. Such instances, however, are rare for series conducted before 1955. In the more typical case, the film badge results do not account for the participant's complete exposure and doses are reconstructed, if a reconstruction has been requested.

When the badge records are available, the results of the separate badge readings are itemized in the database, along with the corresponding dates and identifiers for each badge. The corresponding identifiers provide a link to the badges stored at Reynolds Electrical and Engineering Company (REECo) in Las Vegas, Nevada. Following this variable-length record, which accounts for the separate dose contributions, the estimated total gamma dose assigned to a person is given as the sum across badges entered for each series. In this way, the database allows entry of separate badge doses as well as a total dose for all external gamma dose contributions within each of the series in which that person has participated. When a dose reconstruction has been carried out, the reconstructed doses are stored in the same manner, accounting for interval-specific and total doses.

No uncertainty estimate is given and there is no data field for upper or lower bounds on the estimated total dose. Although data fields for the internal dose estimates exist in the NTPR database, most individuals do not have internal dose estimates entered into these fields.

As described earlier, individual records contained in the dose field are also accompanied by three fields explaining how the dose was derived (Appendix F): data source, dose explanation, and dosimetry type. The dosimetry type field has 55 numeric codes for different methods of dose assignment, including, for example, "#20 — no dose assigned,"

"#23 — extremity TLD dose assigned by investigation," and "#55 — exposure assigned to cohort member based on more than another cohort film badge, wearer unknown." In this field, there are also alphabetic codes that indicate the minimum detection level (MDL) for the specific type of film badge used. These possible MDLs range from 10 mrem to 120 mrem. It is not clear whether this information on the MDL is ever provided.

Ambiguities in interpreting the dose data may arise because of missing information in the NTPR database. Appendix G illustrates such an example by using a case presented to the Working Group at its site visit to JAYCOR. In this case, four separate film badge readings are listed for the veteran's participation in Operation CASTLE. It is not clear, however, whether these readings were based on individual or cohort badges, since the dosimetry type field (T1) is left blank for all four badge readings. After reviewing the SAIC dose reconstruction report, however, it became clear that the first of the four readings is identified as a cohort badge reading, whereas the remaining three readings are identified as being individual badges issued to the veteran. In cohort badging, film badges were often issued to representative personnel in units with common activities and equivalent relationships to the radiation environment.

It is important to note, however, that when the dosimetry type code corresponds to 34, "exposure assigned to cohort based on average of several film badges," it is difficult to know exactly what dose assignment method was used. Sometimes, a dose was assigned that is equal to the mean of the cohort badges plus two standard deviations (97.5 percentile). This is in accord with the methods to be used for assigning radiation doses as described in the *Federal Register* (50 FR 42258 October 21, 1985). In other instances, the average dose was assigned. Because these instances are not identifiable in the database, it cannot be determined whether the former method was chosen or whether the average was actually assigned. This ambiguity is further complicated by the fact that summing across a number of 97.5 percentile levels yields a total dose that is at an even higher percentile.

Although the dose data have been updated over time, the history of dose estimate changes is not traceable in the NTPR database, since only the latest dose assignment for each period of exposure is maintained, and the reason for change is not specified. This is illustrated in Appendix G. It may be possible to trace the dose assignment history by using transaction record tapes maintained by REECo since 1988. Even if full transaction records were to exist, however, the policy decisions on which the changes were based may not be available.

The NTPR database includes a field for occupational code of the participant at the time of a test series. However, it appears that this field is usually vacant. Even after a dose reconstruction that includes use of an occupational title and grade, the corresponding code is not always entered in the database (see Appendices G and H). The NTPR database does not contain the veterans' military specialty codes for the period of participation in weapons tests, for subsequent periods of service, or at the time of discharge. Such information would be important for tracking potential occupational exposures to radiation subsequent to series exposure. For example, it is highly likely that veterans who were involved in radiological sciences during their service have continued to be involved as civilians in occupations related to nuclear power or radiological sciences. In those cases, subsequent radiation doses may outweigh the doses received during weapons tests.

Film Badge Dosimetry

The principal source of film badge information is the REECo master file located in Las Vegas. In reviewing the badge information, the Working Group found that correction factors recommended by the previous NRC committees had not been applied consistently to NTPR dose assignments. The two NRC committees, (1985a, 1989) noted that film badge readings were biased high for actual exposures. It was also noted that the deep dose equivalent in rem would be only 0.8 to 0.9 of the true exposure in roentgens (NRC, 1989). The latter NRC committee had recommended corrections for overall bias ranging from 1.1 to 1.4, that is the badge readings should be divided by these correction factors to obtain the best estimate. The DNA did not adopt these correction factors to modify film badge results. Instead, it has established policy that "Film badge readings expressed in terms of roentgens (R) or its subunits shall be converted directly to dose equivalent in rem, i.e. 1.0 roentgen equals 1.0 rem. This factor allows an unequivocal traceability of film badge doses directly to source records containing film badge readings. Conversion to deep-dose equivalent and the associated bias factor (1.3) shall not be applied" (NTPR, 1992).

In the case of Operation REDWING, the NRC (1989) recommended no bias correction for environmentally damaged badges. By utilizing new findings on the REDWING badges, however, DNA concluded that "Judging from recent dose reconstructions and film badge analysis by SAIC, it is evident that the NAS guidance is incomplete and appropriate action must he taken to portray REDWING doses more accurately" ("Analysis of REDWING Film Badges," RARP/NTPR memorandum, 9 October 1992). Subsequent to this policy decision, however, DNA decided that it will revise REDWING film badge doses only as required to support veterans applying for compensation from the Department of Veterans Affairs.

The correction factors recommended by the NRC Committee (1989) do not account for additional biases introduced when an unbadged individual's dose is derived from cohort badge data. Originally, badging was not done in order to estimate individual exposures for epidemiologic purposes, but rather to verify that radiation safety limits were not exceeded. During the GREENHOUSE and UPSHOT-KNOTHOLE series, and to some degree in the CASTLE series, cohort badging was often used to represent the entire unit or group. Dosimeters, however, also tended to be assigned to radiation monitors and others who were expected to receive the highest doses.

According to the DNA, the number of participants whose dose data were derived from film badges varied substantially for the Five-Series participants (see Table 1). The overall fraction of individual Five-Series participants with doses based on film badge data is approximately one-half. This number of badged personnel, however, can be misleading. The primary reason is that it does not represent the number of participants who actually wore undamaged badges during their entire period of exposure, for whom good dosimetry data can be obtained.

TABLE 1. Description of Approximate Numbers of Participants, Number of Personnel Issued Personal Dosimeters (film badges), and Dosimeter Correction Factors as Determined by the NRC (1989).

Test Series	No. of Participants[a]	No. of Badged Participants[a]	Dosimeter Correction (B) and Uncertainty (K) Factors[b]
GREENHOUSE (1951, Pacific)	7,723	2,317 (30%)	B = 1.4; K = 2.0
UPSHOT-KNOTHOLE (1953, Nevada)	17,062	2,282 (13%)	B = 1.1; K = 1.5
CASTLE (1954, Pacific)	13,958	8,113 (58%)	B = 1.3; K = 2.1
REDWING (1956, Pacific)	13,540	11,044 (82%)	B = 1.3; K = 1.5
PLUMBBOB (1957, Nevada)	12,938	10,243 (79%)	B = 1.3; K = 1.5
Total	65,221	33,999 (52%)	

[a] NTPR data distributed to the Working Group by DNA on 12 April 1994.
[b] B = estimated bias correction (divide by this number to obtain the corrected dose). K = estimated geometric uncertainty factor, as recommended by NRC (1989). 95% confidence limits on a single badge dose can be obtained by multiplying the badge reading, after correcting for bias, by (1/K) and K.

The following reasons explain why these film badge data would not be a suitable subset of NTPR dosimetry information for use in epidemiologic studies:

- an undetermined number of these badges (REDWING) may have been environmentally damaged by high temperature, high humidity, water or light leaks (NRC, 1989);

- some of these individuals may have been assigned doses based upon cohort badging (CASTLE, GREENHOUSE, and UPSHOT-KNOTHOLE);
- some film badges lacked adequate identifying information to uniquely link them to an individual (CASTLE);
- although an individual may have been badged in one series, he may have participated in other series for which he was not badged;
- in some instances, the dose is based solely on the individual's medical records, which listed film badge doses without clear explanation as to whether they covered the person's entire exposure period; and
- for certain series (GREENHOUSE), only one date (e.g., date of issue) was recorded for film badges, so that the actual interval of exposure is unknown.

Reconstructed doses

When film badge dose data were not available or were incomplete, or when there was reason to believe that these data did not adequately characterize the actual exposure, alternative approaches were sometimes used to estimate doses. All approaches commonly involve the investigation of individual or group activities and their relationship to the radiation environment. First, if it was apparent that personnel were not present in the radiation environment — that is, personnel were far distant from the nuclear test(s) and did not experience fallout or enter the fallout area — and had no other potential for exposure, then the assigned dose was zero. Second, if some members of a group had film badge readings and others who did not wear film badges had a common relationship with the radiation environment, NTPR used cohort badging to derive individual doses for unbadged personnel. Third, when sufficient badge readings or a common relationship to the radiation exposure did not exist, doses were sometimes reconstructed. Consistent application of these methods to assign doses did not begin, however, until after 1987, when the DNA consolidated the individual service databases.

For example, doses to typical crew members on ships may have been reconstructed from radiation survey measurements and assumptions of time spent topside and below decks (Thomas et al., 1982). In some instances, different approaches were taken. In the case of UPSHOT-KNOTHOLE, observers without badges were assigned the highest dose measured among the observers who wore badges, regardless of how long they were

There was an apparent lack of consistency between the Army and Navy approaches in assigning reconstructed doses. When the DNA consolidated the service NTPR teams, the Navy provided documentation of the level of confidence associated with assigned doses, whereas the Army did not. The Working Group found no Air Force documentation on the rationale or confidence level for assigned doses.

Most of the reconstructed doses were based on units or groups, but there were approximately 560 cases of some 70,000 Five-Series participants for whom the doses were reconstructed on an individual basis. Once an atomic veteran has developed cancer and he or his surrogates have filed a claim for health or death benefits, a set of institutional responses is set in motion. Typically, and especially if he developed a radiogenic form of cancer such as leukemia, the DNA requests that SAIC undertake an individualized dose reconstruction. Because the individualized dose reconstructions cost about $3,000 each, the process is generally only carried out if there is a specific institutional or legal need for a refined estimate. All periods of potential exposure are identified and examined to verify as accurately as possible the duty assignment and actual locations that the veteran claimed. Film badge data are reviewed for validity. Sufficient information might have been obtained from these additional verification steps to allow a more rigorous dose assignment method than was possible for a unit- or group-based reconstruction. Thus, by filing a claim for which a reconstruction is needed, a participant may be assigned a dose that is derived differently from the one he would have had, had he not filed a claim. The possibility of this type of differential dose assignment was a significant concern to the Working Group. Because the original dose assigned by a unit-based reconstruction may not be recoverable once an individualized dose has been calculated, one cannot revert to any set of dose estimates that can be assumed to be based on a methodology that is comparable for those who filed a claim for a radiogenic cancer and those who did not.

The Working Group attempted to quantify possible bias in the Five-Series dose data that could have resulted from different treatment of those who had individualized reconstructions and those who did not. This was done by comparing the dose entered in the data file for the 1985 Five Series Study (NRC, 1985b) with that in the current data file for all participants whose name had been referred to SAIC for an individualized dose reconstruction and for a comparison group of participants who had not had an individualized reconstruction. Participants with individualized reconstructions were more likely than those without to have had their doses modified between 1985 and 1994. In both individualized and nonindividualized groups, when there was a change in the assigned dose it was much more likely to be an increase than a decrease.

When individuals whose doses did not change over time were eliminated from consideration, no differences were found in the pattern of changes in dose between the individualized and nonindividualized groups. That is, between these two groups, no difference was detected in the proportion of participants who fell into categories defined by whether their doses went down, went up by a little (up to 1 rem), or went up by a lot (more than 1 rem). Thus, for those individuals whose dose *did* change, it did not appear to make a difference whether they received an individual reconstruction or not. This suggests that the individualized dose reconstruction methodology was not systematically biased relative to the generic "cleaning" of the data.

These findings do not, however, allay one of the Working Group's most serious concerns over differential dose assignment — that individualized doses could have experienced a significantly different pattern of change than nonindividualized doses. Those with an individualized dose were much more likely than those without to have had their dose revised upward. Such a differential pattern could bias any dose-response analysis if cancer cases are more likely than noncases to have an individualized dose reconstruction. Further details of this assessment are given in Appendix I.

In reconstructing doses, the radiation environment was characterized in time and space, as were the activities of the unit or group. The physical models used by SAIC have been calibrated to the dose data that were collected as part of the detonation experiments, along fixed radials (at the Nevada Test Site), or on ships (at the Pacific Proving Grounds), or at fixed locations on the islands. For periods of participation that were not captured by the individual's personnel dosimetry (usually badging), the external gamma dose is calculated at SAIC by applying the computer model to integrate the time-dependent dose rate over the appropriate path, using what is known or can be surmised about the person's movements through space and time and his activities in the radiation environment. When there are qualitative uncertainties (e.g., uncertainty about which ship the person was on during the particular dates), high-sided assumptions are usually employed to resolve them, in order to award the veteran the highest plausible dose.

There are other scenarios under which high-sidedness may be imposed, apparently to give the veteran the benefit of the doubt. For example, a memo from SAIC to NTPR dated September 1993 overturned the dose reconstruction for a participant in GREENHOUSE (1951) in favor of the dose found in a medical record. Quoting from the memo, "...medical record doses for April and May 1951 are 0.25 rem and 0.6 rem ... Because this value is greater than the sum of his film badge dose for 8–13 April (0.095 R) and his reconstructed dose for 14 April to 28 May (0.212 rem) it is retained as the veteran's dose of record while he was in CABILDO from 8 April to 28 May."

Ideally, reconstructed doses include calculations of doses from internal (inhaled) radioactivity, based on duration of direct exposure to airborne fallout and/or to resuspended particles during activities in contaminated areas. Even though the assumptions of airborne concentrations of respirable particles appear to be exaggerated, and calculations are deliberately high-sided (as noted in some of the individual records examined by the Working Group), the internal dose contributions to total dose are generally negligible and would not significantly affect the lifetime doses that would be used in an epidemiologic study.

The DNA documented the methods currently being used by NTPR to estimate doses (Schaeffer, 1993). This compilation was provided to the Working Group for its considerations.

CONCLUSIONS

Based on its findings, the Working Group concluded the following for each of the evaluation criteria.

Consistency in the Technical Approach

The NTPR database reflects numerous types of inconsistencies that compromise its reliability as a basis for epidemiologic study. There was an apparent lack of consistency between the Army and Navy approaches in assigning reconstructed doses. There have been irreversible biases in dose assignments introduced as a matter of policy, but these policies have not been consistent over the life of the NTPR database. Because of these policy changes, repeated dose reconstructions for the same individual do not always agree, but the reasons for the discrepancies and the extent of the bias are not readily apparent. Although there is anecdotal evidence that individual doses may have been greatly underestimated in individual cases, the overall tendency may have been to overestimate both external and internal doses.

Nondifferential Dose Assignment

Dose assignment methods applied to self-selected cases may have differed systematically from those applied to unit-based reconstructions, as additional steps are generally taken in self-selected cases to verify their activities in order to carefully estimate their exposure. This could seriously compromise a dose-response analysis. For example, suppose that doses assigned to self-selected cancer cases tend to be lower than those assigned to others who did not file a claim. This could conceivably occur because original high-siding applied to the unit-based reconstructions is generally removed in the cases of individualized reconstruction. In this instance, the form of the dose-response could be seriously distorted. Using information contained in the current NTPR database, it appears possible that the individualized reconstructions for cancer cases may tend to yield higher doses (Appendix I).

Quality Assurance

The NTPR database has been subject to only limited quality control. There has been little peer review of the methods used and of the actual dose assignments. There is no evidence that dose assignments are verified by an independent source other than the NRC committees' general reviews mentioned earlier. The originator of the dose reconstruction estimates (SAIC) did not have final responsibility for the data actually entered in the JAYCOR database, and, in many instances, dose estimates were adjusted by representatives of the armed services without retrievable documentation or notification of those who initially performed the dose estimates.

Documentation of methods used to assign doses in the NTPR database and documentation of individual doses are inadequate. Changes made to the database are not documented by date and reason, and the old dose data are not preserved in the NTPR database when replaced by updated estimates.

Overall, the Working Group felt that documentation of both methods and individual dose assignments in the NTPR database was not sufficiently precise to permit its use for epidemiology.

Uncertainty Analysis

Although uncertainties have been determined for film badge readings, uncertainty analysis applied to estimated doses lacks comprehensiveness and is not state of the art. For example, uncertainties are not being estimated for error associated with using one member's film reading to infer a dose for another subject who did not wear a badge. No uncertainty estimates for the reconstructed doses are entered into the NTPR database.

In summary, the Working Group concludes that the NTPR dose data are not suitable for dose-response analysis in epidemiology. This conclusion is based on the fact that the NTPR dose data were developed primarily for the purpose of ensuring appropriate follow-up for participating veterans and hence and do not meet standards acceptable for their use in epidemiologic research. The Working Group believes, based on its review, that comprehensive dose reconstructions may be feasible for a limited subset of veterans who participated in the above ground nuclear test program. If doses on this population are required for epidemiologic purposes, they should be recalculated according to the following fundamental principles:

- An *a priori* methodology should be established for the dose reconstruction. The methodology should identify mathematical models to be applied, distributions of parameters, and basic assumptions anticipated in dose analysis.
- The objective of the reconstruction should be to derive a "best estimate" of dose with associated uncertainty.
- Doses should be assigned, to the greatest extent possible, with a system that will ensure consistency and minimize subjectivity.
- Uncertainties should be determined by applying state of the art techniques that incorporate all possible sources of bias and parameter variability.
- The dose assignment method should account for doses to specific organs of interest.

- The dose assignment procedure should incorporate plans for quality assurance, including documentation of methods, testing of models used, and verification of data processing.
- Doses should be assigned without knowledge of subjects' health status or previous dose assignments.

Sincerely,

Clark W. Heath, Jr., M.D.
Chairman
Committee on the Mortility of Military Personnel
Present at Atmospheric Texts of Nuclear Weapons

John E. Till, Ph.D.
Chairman
Dosimetry Working Group

REFERENCES

Defense Nuclear Agency. "For the Record — A History of the Nuclear Test Personnel Review, 1978–1986" ; 1986

50 Federal Register 42258; 21 October 1985 .

Flor WJ and Goetz JL. "DoD Experience with Dose Reconstructions for Atmospheric Test Veterans." Presented at the Environmental Radiation and Public Policy Symposium, Las Vegas, Nevada; October 1991 .

National Research Council. *Review of the Methods Used to Assign Radiation Doses to Service Personnel at Nuclear Weapons Tests.* Washington, D.C., National Academy Press , 1985a .

National Research Council. *Mortality of Nuclear Weapons Test Participants.* Washington, D.C. , National Academy Press , 1985b .

National Research Council. *Film Badge Dosimetry in Atmospheric Nuclear Tests.* Washington, D.C. , National Academy Press , 1989 .

Nuclear Test Personnel Review. Policy Note 02-92 , Defense Nuclear Agency RARP ; 6 July 1992 .

Schaeffer DM. Defense Nuclear Agency. Compilation of Dose Reconstruction Methodology ; 3 December 1993 .

Schaeffer DM. Defense Nuclear Agency. Presentation to the Dosimetry Working Group ; April 1994 .

Thomas C , et al. , "Analysis of Radiation Exposure for Shipyard Naval Personnel, Operation GREENHOUSE," Science Applications International Corporation 83-874-WA ; 30 July 1982 .

APPENDIXES

A

Background of the Five Series Study and the Study Committee Roster

From 1946 through 1962, the U.S. government conducted more than 230 atmospheric tests of nuclear weapons, mainly at the Nevada Test Site and at the Pacific Proving Ground. It is estimated that some 220,000 DoD personnel, both military and civilian, participated in these tests.

In 1979 the Centers for Disease Control published a report* noting an apparent increase in leukemia among the participants present at shot SMOKY, which was detonated in Nevada in 1957. In 1985, the Medical Follow-up Agency (MFUA) of the National Academy of Sciences reported the results of a study of mortality of more than 49,000 military participants attending five nuclear weapon test series, including shot SMOKY. The study reported no consistent, statistically significant evidence of an increase in mortality from any disease other than leukemia among participants at SMOKY. In 1989, MFUA learned from the Defense Nuclear Agency (DNA) that the cohort of atomic veterans on which MFUA based its 1985 study contained misclassification errors. Subsequent investigations by the General Accounting Office and the Office of Technology Assessment concluded that the changes in participant numbers and dose estimates were large enough to require that the study be redone. Subsequent to these reports, MFUA was asked to redo the 1985 study.

The principal purpose of this study is to ascertain whether mortality from leukemia, other cancers, or other diseases has occurred at a higher rate among participants at atmospheric nuclear weapon tests including SMOKY compared with a similar group of veterans who were not participants. This second follow-up study will utilize updated participant identification and radiation exposure data provided by DNA for the same five series of nuclear tests. To conduct the current study, the IOM has established a committee of 10 members representing a range of expertise in epidemiology, biostatistics, radiation biology, radiation medicine, military records, and health physics.

---

*Center for Disease *Control, Leukemia among persons present at an atmospheric nuclear test (SMOKY)*. MMWR 28:361-362, 1979.

Committee to Study the Mortality of Military Personnel Present at Atmospheric Tests of Nuclear Weapons

CHAIRMAN

Clark W. Heath, Jr., M.D.

Vice President for Epidemiology and Surveillance Research

American Cancer Society

Atlanta, GA

Harvey Checkoway, Ph.D.
Professor
Departments of Environmental Health and Epidemiology
University of Washington
Seattle, WA

Richard J. M. Fry, M.D.
Consultant
Oak Ridge National Laboratory
Biology Division
Oak Ridge TN

Samuel Hellman, M.D. (IOM)
A.N. Pritzker Distinguished Service Professor
The Department of Radiation and Cellular Oncology
The University of Chicago
Chicago, IL

Elaine Ron, Ph.D.
Epidemiologist
Radiation Epidemiology Branch
National Institutes of Health
National Cancer Institute
Bethesda, MD

William G. Seibert, M.A.
Senior Archivist
National Personnel Records Center
St. Louis, MO

John E. Till, Ph.D.
President
Radiological Assessments Corporation
Neeses, SC

Clarice R. Weinberg, Ph.D.
Mathematical Statistician
Program of Environmental Biology and Medicine
National Institute of Environmental Health Sciences
Research Triangle Park, NC

STAFF

Richard N. Miller, M.D., MFUA Director
J. Christopher Johnson, Ph.D., Study Director
Erin M. Bell, M.S., Research Associate
Harriet Crawford, Manager of Data Management Team
Chiquita M. H. Benson, B.S., Programmer Analyst
Alexander Saenger, B.S., Programmer Analyst
Sylvia McKinnis, Mgr. St. Louis Office
Mary Juman, Records Assistant Denise Parker - Coder Abstractor
Pamela Ramey-McCray, Project Assistant

Former Committee Members and Staff

David G. Hoel, Ph.D. (Committee *Chair*)
H. Rodney Withers, M.D., Ph.D. (Committee Member)
Christopher P. Howson, Ph.D. (Staff)
Youn K. Shim, Ph.D. (Staff)

B

Dosimetry Working Group Roster

Committee to Study the Mortality of Military Personnel Present at Atmospheric Tests of Nuclear Weapons

Dosimetry Working Group

John E. Till, Ph.D., Chairman *
President, Radiological *Assessments* Corporation
Neeses, SC
F. Owen Hoffman, Ph.D.
SENES of Oak Ridge, Inc.
Oak Ridge, TN
Keith J. Schiager, Ph.D. **
Department of Radiological Health
University of Utah
Salt Lake City, UT
John Taschner
Los Alamos National Laboratory
Los Alamos, NM
Clarice R. Weinberg, Ph.D. *
Program of Environmental Biology and Medicine
National Institute of Environmental
Health Sciences
Research Triangle Park, NC

* Member of the Committee
** Member of the Crossroads Study Committee

C

Background of the NTPR Program

In 1978, shortly after DNA became the DoD executive agency for matters pertaining to participants of DoD personnel in the atmospheric nuclear tests, DNA established the NTPR program. The NTPR program was responsible for the following tasks (DNA, 1986):

- developing a history of every atmospheric nuclear event that involved DoD personnel;
- identifying the radiation monitoring control policies and procedures that were in effect;
- identifying DoD personnel involved in the atmospheric nuclear tests and providing estimates of their radiation exposures;
- making this information available for scientific review and appraisal; and
- handling Congressional and public affairs matters.

Initially, DNA directed each individual military service to conduct the NTPR research on its own personnel and to develop its own database for the NTPR. In an effort to ensure that the information was collected consistently across services, DNA specified data fields for each of the service NTPR databases. However, the DNA did not specify to the services how the available data were to be used in assigning doses. In 1987, DNA consolidated the individual NTPR teams into a single team and merged the data from the separate services.

To assist it in executing the NTPR program, DNA employed three contractors: JAYCOR, Science Applications International Corporation (SAIC), and Reynolds Electrical & Engineering Company (REECo) (DNA, 1994, D.M. Schaeffer presentation to the Dosimetry Working Group, April 1994). Historical research and database services were provided by JAYCOR. Its findings are used to verify participation of veterans in the atmospheric nuclear weapon tests and to provide the historical basis for dose reconstructions. It also maintains the NTPR database that documents veterans' participation, VA claims history, most recently assigned dose and other related information. Dose reconstruction services were provided by SAIC using historical information provided by JAYCOR. The "master" nuclear testing dosimetry database, originally developed for the Department of Energy, is maintained by REECo (Flor and Goetz, 1990).

The process of identifying participants and estimating their doses is a continuing one. Participant rosters and exposure assessments are updated as federal criteria for inclusion evolve and as additional historical records are found providing new unit names or other information used for dose assignment. When DNA assigns or changes a veteran's dose, the new dose is entered into the NTPR database and is also forwarded to REECo, which updates the veteran's dose in its database. While the NTPR database has kept only the most recent dose estimate, REECo has retained transaction records since 1988 for previously assigned doses (personal communication, DM Schaeffer, DNA, 31 May 1994).

D

Background Materials Provided to the Working Group Prior to its First Meeting

- A "Dose Reconstruction Methodology" binder provided by the DNA. Contained in this document is the FEDERAL REGISTER notice of 21 October 1985, "Guidance for the Determination and Reporting of Nuclear Radiation Dose for DoD Participants in the Atmospheric Nuclear Test Program." The binder also contains excerpts from relevant documents describing the methodologies for reconstructing external doses based on field surveys and internal doses from resuspension and inhalation of fallout.
- "DoD Experience with Dose Reconstructions for Atmospheric Test Veterans"
- "Analysis of Radiation Exposure for Shipyard Naval Personnel, Operation GREENHOUSE"
- "Neutron Exposure for DoD Nuclear Test Personnel"

E

NTPR Database Fields Relevant to this Review *

"ID INFORMATION"	
LAST TRANSACTION —	date of last record update
OVER 5 REM —	indicates that the total dose exceeds 5 rem in 12 consecutive months
RADIOGENIC CLAIM —	indicates a VA claim for a radiogenic cancer, with claim number, ICD-8 codes, VA Regional Office and Court of Veterans Appeals indicated in the following fields.
"PERS INFORMATION"	
DEATH IND —	indicates the individual has died; subsequent fields indicate date and cause.
CANCER IND —	indicates the individual has cancer.
"CORR INFORMATION"	
CORR CODE —	Column 1 contains code letter for type of response: A: File A letter C: Congressional letter F: Freedom of Information I: Individual V: VA O: Other

*An example of an NTPR Participant Information File is shown in APPENDIX G-1

"SERIES INFORMATION"	
This section contains general information about the participant's status during a specific test series.	
PAR CAT —	participant category code
OCCUP —	occupation code at time of series (usually vacant)
"UNIT INFORMATION"	
This section indicates the specific unit assignment and inclusive dates of participation in the test series, as well as the individual's permanent unit assignment.	
"BADGED DOSES"	
BADGED DATE —	contains start and ending dates for each badge record.
GAMMA —	contains the dose of record (mrem), which is usually thefilm badge reading; the number following the colon indicates the source of the assigned dose.
E1 and E2 —	contain codes for an explanation of the dose assignment.
T1 and T2 —	contain codes that indicate type of dosimetry worn, e.g., "01:34" refers to a "field packet dosimeter" with the source being the "REECo dosimetry primary source documents."
REECo NUM —	is the access number that provides the link to REECo records; this is usually a film packet ID number.
TURN-IN and PROC-DT —	contain dates badges were turned in and processed, but they are usually vacant.
"RECONSTRUCTED DOSES"	
These fields contain information from reconstruction that is similar to badged doses with the following exceptions:	
LOW and HIGH —	indicate the range of possible gamma doses.

CHG-DT —	indicates the date the reconstructed dose was entered in the database.
RECON ID —	identifies the reconstruction documentation by data.
"INTERNAL DOSES"	
BPCD —	indicates the organ receiving the dose shown in the DOSE column.

F

Source Codes for NTPR Data Fields Relevant to this Review Provided by DNA/ JAYCOR

DATA ELEMENT 62-66	
01	FIELD PACKET DOSIMETER
02	TLD
03	POCKET DOSIMETER
04	IN VIVO COUNT
05	WHOLE BODY COUNT
06	BIOASSAY RESULT
07	INVESTIGATION ASSIGNED BY DOSE RATE
08	INVESTIGATION ASSIGNED BY OTHER BADGED PERSON
09	INVESTIGATION ASSIGNED FROM DAMAGED FILM
10	CALCULATED FROM LOCATION
11	CALCULATED FROM FALLOUT
12	CHEMICAL DOSIMETER
13	NRDS PENETRATION-NONPENETRATING DOSIMETRY
14	TLD NEUTRON DOSIMETER
15	NTA FAST NEUTRON FILM PACKET
16	ACCIDENT DOSIMETRY
17	ASSIGNED FROM AIR CONCENTRATION
18	EXTREMITY DOSIMETRY-FILM
19	EXTREMITY DOSIMETRY-TLD
20	NO DOSE ASSIGNED
21	DOSIMETER TYPE UNKNOWN AND/OR DOSIMETER NUMBER ASSIGNED BY REECO (WHEN DOSIMETER NUMBER IS BLANK, AND THERE IS A PERMANENT OR MISSION BADGE DOSE)
22	FILM PACKET DOSIMETER, DOSE ASSIGNED BY INVESTIGATION
23	EXTREMITY TLD DOSE ASSIGNED BY INVESTIGATION
24	NEUTRON TLD, DOSE ASSIGNED BY INVESTIGATION
25	NTA FAST NUETRON FILM, DOSE ASSIGNED BY INVESTIGATION
26	DOSE TYPE UNKNOWN, DOSE ASSIGNED BY INVESTIGATION
27	KODAK FILM WITH "J" AS FIRST POSITION OF FILM NUMBER
28	KODAK FILM WITH "J" AS FIRST POSITION OF FILM NUMBER, DOSE ASSIGNED BY INVESTIGATION
29	DOSE ASSIGNED BY HEALTH PHYSICIST EVALUATION
30	RECONSTRUCTION OF REECO FILM BADGE RECORDS
31	TLD CARD, DOSE ASSIGNED BY INVESTIGATION
32	EXPOSURE ASSIGNED TO COHORT FROM COHORT MEMBER FILM BADGE

33	EXPOSURE ASSIGNED TO COHORT BASED ON AVERAGE OF SHIP EXPOSURE
34	EXPOSURE ASSIGNED TO COHORT BASED ON AVERAGE OF SEVERAL FILM BADGES
35	EXPOSURE ASSIGNED TO COHORT BASED ON "LESS THAN ANOTHER COHORT BADGE EXPOSURE"
36	EXPOSURE ASSIGNED TO COHORT BASED ON "MORE THAN ANOTHER COHORT BADGE EXPOSURE"
37	RESIDUAL OR ADDITIONAL EXPOSURE IN FINAL REPORTS, NOT FOUND IN DOSIMETRY SOURCE DOCUMENTS
38	DOSE ASSIGNED TO COHORT BASED ON HIGH EXPOSURE OF SHIP
39	EVIDENCE INDICATES PARTICIPANT DID NOT WEAR ASSIGNED FILM BADGE
40	EXPOSURE ASSIGNED TO COHORT BADGE WEARER FROM COHORT FILM BADGE.
41	EXPOSURE ASSIGNED TO COHORT BADGE WEARER BASED ON AVERAGE OF SHIP EXPOSURE.
42	EXPOSURE ASSIGNED TO COHORT BADGE WEARER BASED ON AVERAGE OF SEVERAL FILM BADGES.
43	EXPOSURE ASSIGNED TO COHORT MEMBER FROM COHORT FILM BADGE, WEARER UNKNOWN.
44	EXPOSURE ASSIGNED TO COHORT MEMBER BASED ON AVERAGE OF SHIP EXPOSURE, WEARER UNKNOWN.
45	EXPOSURE ASSIGNED TO COHORT MEMBER BASED ON AVERAGE OF SEVERAL FILM BADGES, WEARER UNKNOWN.
46	EXPOSURE ASSIGNED TO COHORT BADGE WEARER BASED ON LESS THAN ANOTHER COHORT FILM BADGE
47	EXPOSURE ASSIGNED TO COHORT BADGE WEARER BASED ON MORE THAN ANOTHER COHORT FILM BADGE
48	OPTICAL DENSITY USED ERRONEOUSLY TO DETERMINE EXPOSURES
49	NO DOSE ASSIGNED TO COHORT BADGE MEMBER
50	NO DOSE ASSIGNED TO COHORT BADGE WEARER
51	NO DOSE ASSIGNED TO COHORT MEMBER, BADGE WEARER UNKNOWN.

52	DOSE ASSIGNED TO COHORT BADGE WEARER BASED ON HIGH EXPOSURE OF SHIP.
53	DOSE ASSIGNED TO COHORT MEMBER BASED ON HIGH EXPOSURE OF SHIP
54	DOSE ASSIGNED TO COHORT MEMBER BASED ON LESS THAN ANOTHER COHORT FILM BADGE, WEARER UNKNOWN
55	EXPOSURE ASSIGNED TO COHORT MEMBER BASED ON MORE THAN ANOTHER COHORT FILM BADGE, WEARER UNKNOWN
MA	FILM BADGE: PROCESSING MDL = 10 MR
MB	FILM BADGE: PROCESSING MDL = 15 MR
MC	FILM BADGE: PROCESSING MDL = 20 MR
MD	FILM BADGE: PROCESSING MDL = 25 MR
ME	FILM BADGE: PROCESSING MDL = 30 MR
MF	FILM BADGE: PROCESSING MDL = 35 MR
MG	FILM BADGE: PROCESSING MDL = 40 MR
MH	FILM BADGE: PROCESSING MDL = 45 MR
MI	FILM BADGE: PROCESSING MDL = 50 MR
MJ	FILM BADGE: PROCESSING MDL = 55 MR
MK	FILM BADGE: PROCESSING MDL = 60 MR
ML	FILM BADGE: PROCESSING MDL = 65 MR
MM	FILM BADGE: PROCESSING MDL = 70 MR
MN	FILM BADGE: PROCESSING MDL = 75 MR
MO	FILM BADGE: PROCESSING MDL = 80 MR
MP	FILM BADGE: PROCESSING MDL = 85 MR
MO	FILM BADGE: PROCESSING MDL = 90 MR
MR	FILM BADGE: PROCESSING MDL = 95MR
MS	FILM BADGE: PROCESSING MDL = 100 MR
MT	FILM BADGE: PROCESSING MDL = 105 MR
MU	FILM BADGE: PROCESSING MDL = 110 MR
MV	FILM BADGE: PROCESSING MDL = 115 MR
MW	FILM BADGE: PROCESSING MDL = 120 MR

DATA ELEMENTS 83-88

A	LOST BADGE
B	LIGHT DAMAGED
C	HEAT DAMAGED
D	PRESSURE DAMAGED
E	FACTORY DAMAGED
F	PROCESSING DAMAGED
G	MEDICAL EXPOSURE
H	NON PERS. OR NON OCCUPATIONAL X-RAY
I	DESTROYED
J	WATER DAMAGED
K	AGE DAMAGED
L	UNDETERMINED DAMAGE
M	MONITORED, NO DOSE ASSIGNED
N	OCCUPATION DAMAGE
O	NON - RETURN
P	PRESENT, BUT NOT MONITORED
Q	RESIDUAL DOSE FROM REECO SOURCE DOCUMENT
R	RECONSTRUCTED
S	ESTIMATED
T	COMBINED (ESTIMATED & ACTUAL)
U	PRESENT, BUT MONITORING UNKNOWN
V	MULTIPLE BADGES WORN/HIGHEST DOSE ASSIGNED
W	MULTIPLE BADGES WORN/LOWEST DOSE NOT ASSIGNED
X	DOSE ASSIGNED BY INVESTIGATION
Y	OCCUPATION X-RAY
Z	BADGE ASSIGNED TO EQUIPMENT ONLY
1	NEUTRON MONITORED POSITIVE DOSE INCLUDED IN GAMMA DOSE FIELD
2	MULTIPLE BADGES WORN, AVERAGE DOSE ASSIGNED
3	DOSIMETER ISSUED, NO RESULTS AVAILABLE

4	DOSE RESULTS AVAILABLE, ISSUE DATE AND/OR RETURN OR PROCESS DATE INFORMATION NOT AVAILABLE
5	EXPOSURE RESULTS LESS THAN 50 MREM MAY BE QUESTIONABLE
6	BASED ON MEDICAL RECORD REMARK INDICATING NO EXPOSURE; FILM BADGE NOT USED AS BASIS FOR EXPOSURE
7	THE NET OPTICAL DENSITY OR PROBIT DENSITY IS UNKNOWN, THE GAMMA EXPOSURE IS REPORTED AS A “LESS THAN” VALUE OR “ZERO” IN THE SOURCE DOCUMENT
8	NAME APPEARS ON BLANK DOSIMETRY CARD, MAY NOT HAVE BEEN PARTICIPANT
9	EXPOSURE ASSIGNED FROM ANOTHER PERSON'S FILM BADGE
0 (zero)	FILM BADGE DAMAGED BY RADIOACTIVE CONTAMINATION
=	THE NET OPTICAL DENSITY OR PROBIT DENSITY IS REPORTED AS ZERO, THE GAMMA EXPOSURE IS REPORTED AS A “LESS THAN” VALUE OR “ZERO” IN THE SOURCE DOCUMENT
+	THE NET OPTICAL DENSITY OR PROBIT DENSITY IS REPORTED AS A POSITIVE VALUE, THE GAMMA EXPOSURE IS REPORTED AS A “LESS THAN” VALUE OR “ZERO” IN THE SOURCE DOCUMENT
#	THE GAMMA EXPOSURE IS REPORTED AS A “LESS THAN” VALUE OR “ZERO” IN THE SOURCE DOCUMENT, BUT THERE WAS NO OPPORTUNITY FOR EXPOSURE
A1	NOT PRESENT FOR ENTIRE COHORT BADGE PERIOD
A2	COMBINED (ACTUAL AND RECONSTRUCTED)
A3	ENVIRONMENTAL DAMAGE
A4	READING FROM HIGH RANGE BADGE
A5	POSTING ERROR
A6	NET OPTICAL DENSITY OR PROBIT DENSITY IS REPORTED “ZERO” THE GAMMA EXPOSURE IS REPORTED AS A POSITIVE VALUE IN THE SOURCE DOCUMENT

UNOFFICIAL COPY

Change October 1, 1993

DATA ELEMENT 99

01	LEXINGTON BLUE GRASS MICROFILM
02	MORNING REPORTS
03	SECURITY CLEARANCE FORMS
04	ORDERS
05	SECURITY ROSTERS
06	DISCHARGE PAPERS
07	MEDICAL RECORDS
08	LETTERS AND PHONE CALLS OTHER THAN JAYCOR
09	LETTERS AND PHONE CALLS - JAYCOR
10	GENERAL SERVICES ADMINISTRATION (GSA) REGISTRY # 1
11	VETERANS ADMINISTRATION (VA)
12	REYNOLDS ELECTRICAL & ENGINEERING COMPANY (REECO) SECONDARY SOURCE DOCUMENTS
13	CENTER FOR DISEASE CONTROL (CDC)
14	INTERNAL REVENUE SERVICE (IRS)
15	SCIENCE APPLICATIONS INTERNATIONAL CORP. [SAIC)
16	NATIONAL ACADEMY OF SCIENCES (NAS)
17	THE ADJUTANT GENERAL (TAG)
18	NAVY
19	AIR FORCE
20	MARINE CORPS
21	COAST GUARD
22	ARMY
23	JAYCOR
24	DNA ANALYSIS OF DATA
25	DEFENSE NUCLEAR AGENCY (DNA)
26	DASIAC
27	MUSTER ROLLS (NAVY)
28	DECK LOG LIST OF OFFICERS (NAVY)
29	DAILY DECK LOG (NAVY)
30	BUMED (NAVY)
31	MULTIPLE SOURCES

32	UNIT/PERSONNEL DIARY
33	GENERATED ID NUMBER
34	REECO DOSIMETRY PRIMARY SOURCE DOCUMENTS
35	DISCHARGE REVIEW BOARD
36	ARMY COUNCIL OF REVIEW BOARDS
37	ARMY BOARD FOR CORRECTION OF MILITARY RECORDS
38	NATIONAL PERSONNEL RECORD CENTER (NPRC)
39	RESERVE COMPONENT PERSONNEL ADMINISTRATION CENTER (RCPAC)
40	RETIRED PAY DIVISION - US ARMY FINANCE AND ACCOUNTING CENTER(USAFAC)
41	FEDERAL BUREAU OF INVESTIGATION (FBI)
42	MILITARY PERSONNEL CENTER (MILPERCEN)
43	AFSWP DOSE LETTER OF 9 JUN 55
44	DEPARTMENT OF ENERGY (DOE)
45	PERSONNEL RECORD
46	DNA/FIELD COMMAND
47	UNITED STATES ARMY MANAGEMENT SYSTEMS SUPPORT AGENCY(USAMSSA)
48	REECO/H&N MICROFILM
49	REECO/SANDIA MICROFILM
50	REECO/LLL SOURCE DOCUMENT
51	REECO/LASL MAGNETIC TAPE
52	AFTER ACTION REPORT
53	LASL RECORDS
54	AEC DOCUMENT
55	DOE NV 185-RADIATION EXPOSURE HISTORY INQUIRY
56	AFSWP DOCUMENTS
57	RESEARCH & DEVELOPMENT BOARD OF D.O.D.
58	EBERLINE INSTRUMENT CORP.
59	REECO DOSIMETRY ISSUE CARD
60	REECO NTS/SSN

61	GENERAL SERVICES ADMINISTRATION (GSA) REGISTRY # 2
62	GENERAL SERVICES ADMINISTRATION (GSA) REGISTRY # 3
63	ORIGINAL SOURCE DATE INCOMPLETE. CHECK SOURCE RECORDS FOR ANY ADDITIONAL INFORMATION.
64	JAYCOR/NUS
65	REECO PAYROLL HISTORY CARDS
70	AVAILABLE EVIDENCE INDICATES PARTICIPANT NOT EXPOSED TO IONIZING RADIATION.
71	GAMMA DOSE ASSIGNED TO PARTICIPANT BASED ON DOSIMETRY RECORDS OF OTHER TEST PARTICIPANTS. PROBABLE DOSE/DOSE RANGE ENTERED AS REMARKS IN BIOASSAY DATA FIELD.
72	DOSE/DOSE RANGE ASSIGNMENT OF PARTICIPANT BASED ON FORMAL DOSE RECONSTRUCTION BY SAIC. PROBABLE DOSE/ DOSE RANGE ENTERED AS REMARK IN BIOASSAY DATA FIELD.
73	DOSE/DOSE RANGE ASSIGNMENT OF PARTICIPANT BASED ON FORMAL DOSE RECONSTRUCTION BY DNA. PROBABLE DOSE/ DOSE RANGE ENTERED AS REMARK IN BIOASSAY DATA FIELD.
74	DOSE/DOSE RANGE ASSIGNMENT OF PARTICIPANT BASED ON FORMAL DOSE RECONSTRUCTION BY NAVY. PROBABLE DOSE/ DOSE RANGE ENTERED AS REMARK IN BIOASSAY DATA FIELD.
75	DOSE/DOSE RANGE ASSIGNMENT OF PARTICIPANT BASED ON FORMAL DOSE RECONSTRUCTION BY AIR FORCE. PROBABLE DOSE/DOSE RANGE ENTERED AS REMARK IN BIOASSAY DATA FIELD.
76	DOSE/DOSE RANGE ASSIGNMENT OF PARTICIPANT BASED ON FORMAL DOSE RECONSTRUCTION BY MARINE CORPS. PROBABLE DOSE/DOSE RANGE ENTERED AS REMARK IN BIOASSAY DATA FIELD.

77	DOSE/DOSE RANGE ASSIGNMENT OF PARTICIPANT BASED ON FORMAL DOSE RECONSTRUCTION BY ARMY. PROBABLE DOSE/ DOSE RANGE ENTERED AS REMARK IN BIOASSAY DATA FIELD.
78	DOSE/DOSE RANGE ASSIGNMENT OF PARTICIPANT BASED ON FORMAL DOSE RECONSTRUCTION. PROBABLE DOSE/DOSE RANGE ENTERED AS REMARK IN BIOASSAY DATA FIELD.
79	NO RECORDED GAMMA DOSE. NO DOSE RECONSTRUCTION PLANNED.
80	NEUTRON DOSE ASSIGNED TO PARTICIPANT BASED ON DOSIMETRY RECORDS OF OTHER TEST PARTICIPANTS. PROBABLE DOSE/DOSE RANGE ENTERED AS REMARK IN BIOASSAY DATA FIELD.
81	DOSIMETER ISSUED. NO RESULTS AVAILABLE.
82	REECO SOURCE DOCUMENT FILM BADGE RECORD - MILITARY MEDICAL RECORDS EXIST AND CANNOT BE PROVEN TO BE IN ERROR.
83	ASSIGNED DOSE RESIDUAL FROM MEDICAL RECORD NOT ACCOUNTED FOR WITH FILM BADGE RECORDS, AND MEDICAL RECORD CANNOT BE PROVEN TO BE IN ERROR.
84	REECO SOURCE DOCUMENT FILM BADGE RECORD - MILITARY MEDICAL RECORD EXISTS AND PROVEN TO BE IN ERROR.
85	FLIGHT LOG
86	MUSTER ROLLS (MARINE CORPS)
87	RECORDS OF THE JUDGE ADVOCATE GENERAL, RG 153 (POWS)
88	RECORDS OF THE PROVOST MARSHAL GENERAL, RG 389 (POWS)
89	RECORDS OF THE ADJUTANT GENERAL'S OFFICE, PHILIPPINE ARCHIVES COLLECTION, RG 407 (POWS)
90	VETERANS ADMINISTRATION POW LIST
91	CRUISE BOOK/UNOFFICIAL UNIT HISTORY
92	SHIP MOVEMENT REPORT

93	ASSIGNED BEGIN DATE FOR FILM BADGE EXPOSURE PERIOD IS BASED ON RESEARCH
94	ASSIGNED END DATE FOR FILM BADGE EXPOSURE PERIOD IS BASED ON RESEARCH
95	GREENHOUSE FILM BADGE DATA SHEET (CTG 3.3)
96	MILITARY SERVICE UNIT HISTORY
97	MILITARY SERVICE UNIT ROSTER
98	ASSIGNED BEGIN AND END DATES FOR FILM BADGE EXPOSURE PERIOD IS BASED ON RESEARCH
99	POST-CROSSROADS SHIPYARD REPORTS (CIVILIAN AND MILITARY)
AA	POSTING DATE NO OTHER DATES AVAILABLE
AB	BADGE NUMBER ON SOURCE DOCUMENT HAS BEEN PROVEN TO BE IN ERROR.
AC	BADGE NUMBER ON SOURCE DOCUMENT UNREADABLE.
AD	ATTACH DATE NOT IN SERIES YEAR RECORDS. APPEARS TO HAVE ATTACHED IN PREVIOUS YEAR. DETACH DATE CORRECT.
AE	DETACH DATE NOT IN SERIES YEAR RECORDS. APPEARS TO HAVE DETACHED IN FOLLOWING YEAR. ATTACH DATE CORRECT.

* Requested by REECO
** Requested by JAYCOR

Defense Nuclear Agency 6801 Telegraph Road Alexandria. Virginia 22310-3398 28 MAR 1994 Reynolds Electrical and Engineering Company, Inc. ATTN: Mr. Tom Bastian

Mail Stop 543

P.O. Box 98521 Las Vegas, Nevada 89193-8521 Dear Mr. Bastian:

We have determined that two new source codes are needed.

AD Attach date not in Series year records. Appears to have attached in previous year. Detach date correct.

AE Detach date not in Series year records. Appears to have detached in following year. Attach date correct.

These codes are needed to indicate to researchers that Series year records have been researched for attach or detach dates. If attach/detach dates are required, it indicates what research has been completed and where to start looking for dates.

Sincerely,

D. M. Schaeffer Program Manager Nuclear Test Personnel Review Radiation Sciences Directorate

G

Example of Film Badge Data (Operation CASTLE)

For a participant in the CASTLE series, four periods of doses obtained from badge data are shown (Appendix G-1 #1). There are no entries to indicate whether these were individual or cohort badges; however, the dose reconstruction (Appendix G-2 #1) indicates that the first of the four was a cohort badge, whereas the other three values were individual badges.

The database includes a small internal dose for this individual. Although the code for the source of this internal dose calculation is shown as ":72," indicating an SAIC dose reconstruction, there is no entry in the last column "CHG-DT" (G-1 #3) to verify that the 8 December 1993 document (G-2) is the basis for the number. Code "19" under "BPCD" (G-1 #4) indicates that this is a dose to the kidneys (G-2 #4).

Appendix G-2 also illustrates the concern of the Working Group with respect to biases in the data. Two statements (G-2 #2 and G-2 #3) refer to high-siding of the internal dose calculation.

G-1

Personal Information Form — Film Badge Data

Operation CASTLE

```
JC14.                          PERSONAL   INFORMATION   FORM                              03-JUN-1994
****************************************************************************************************
ID INFORMATION ------------------------------------- NAVY ------------------- LAST TRANSACTION 94/02/09
MIL S#: [redacted] :07  [redacted] :07        :                :
NAME: [redacted]   [redacted]   [redacted]         :07
ALIAS:                          :
SSN1= [redacted] :07   SSN2=        :
STREET= [redacted]                     FILE A IND= A            RADIOG. CLAIM= X
CITY= [redacted]       STATE= [redacted] OVER 5 REM=           VA CLAIM= [redacted]
COUNTRY=      ZIP= [redacted]   :07    JAYCOR CASE= [redacted]  VA CLAIM ICD= [redacted]
PHONE= [redacted] :09                  REECO ACCT= [redacted]   VA REG. OFF.= [redacted]
                                       DOJ JAYCOR CLAIM=        COVA=
                                       DOJ CLAIM=

NEXT KIN IND=  :     REL=        NAME=
---------------------------------------------- PERS INFORMATION -----------------------------------
LAST GRADE= ET3  :09   CIV TITLE=              ENTRY DATE= [redacted] SEPARATION DATE= [redacted]
BIRTH DATE= [redacted] :07, ADDR= [redacted] , MO :07  COUNTRY=     SEX= M :07
DEATH IND=   :    CAUSE=        :    DATE=        :    CANCER IND= X :11
---------------------------------------------- CORR INFORMATION -----------------------------------
  A    84/04/16
  I    81/11/04
  V    94/01/25
  V    93/06/14
---------------------------------------------- SENIER INFORMATION ---------------------------------
************************************************* CASTLE        :10 *******************************
*   GRADE=ET3 :09            PER CAT=04:07         PAR CAT=   :         OCCUP=              SVC=N  *
****************************************************************************************************
---------------------------------------------- UNIT INFORMATION -----------------------------------
PART= [redacted] :45  54/01/21 - 54/07/25:45 ORG=     :    PERM= [redacted] :45
--- #1 ---------------------------------------- BADGED DOSED --------------------------------------
BADGED_DATE         GAMMA      E1 E2 I1    I2 DOSIM_#   REECO_IAN  SERV_ASN_#  ILUM:IN  PROC:DT  DETB  NEUTRN  CUG:DT
540310-540316:94    000335:34        :        08787:34             [redacted]  :        :        :     :       940107
```

Appendix G-1, Personal Information Form - Film Badge Data Operation Castle, Page 1

```
(Cont.)   [redacted]   CASTLE

------------------------------- BADGED DOSES -------------------------------
BADGED_DATE          GAMMA      E1 E2 I1   I2 DOSIM_#    RECCO_NUM  SERV_ASN_#  TURN-IN  PROC-DT  BETA  NEUTRON  CHG-DT
540331-540331:94     000500:34         :      14903:34              [redacted]      :        :       :      :    940107
540401-540401:94     000245:34         :      14104:34                              :        :       :      :    940107
540404-540404:94     000410:34         :      14110:34                              :        :       :      :    940107

TOTAL GAMMA      =     1490
---------------------------- RECONSTRUCTED DOSES ----------------------------
RECON_DATE        HIGH  GAMMA   LOW     E1 E2 I1   I2 RECCO_NUM  SERV_ASN_#  HIGH  NEUTRON  LOW       CHG-DT  RECON_ID
540119-540228:72        000000     :70        :                  [redacted]                          :    940107  9312081
540119-540725:72                   :          :                               000000             :72  940107  9312081
540301-540309:72        000198     :72        :                                                  :    940107  9312081
540317-540330:72        000135     :72        :                                                  :    940107  9312081
540402-540403:72        000048     :72        :                                                  :    940107  9312081
540405-540725:72        000541     :72        :                                                  :    940107  9312081

TOTAL GAMMA                 =      922
TOTAL NEUTRON               =        0
TOTAL GAMMA + NEUTRON       =      922
TOTAL GAMMA FOR SERIES                 =     2412
TOTAL NEUTRON FOR SERIES               =        0
TOTAL (GAMMA + NEUTRON) FOR SERIES     =     2412
-------------------#2---------#4----------------- INTERNAL DO#3 ------------------------
INTERNAL_DATE     DOSE        I1 RECD  E130  RECCO_NUM   SERV_ASN_#  CHG-DT
54    -54    :72  000028:72      19                      [redacted]

TOTAL ALL GAMMA                        =     2412
TOTAL ALL NEUTRON                      =        0
TOTAL ALL (GAMMA + NEUTRON)            =     2412
```

Appendix G-1, Personal Information Form - Film Badge Data Operation Castle, Page 2

G-2

SAIC Memorandum to RAEM/NTPR

Subject: Radiation Dose Assessment for <NAME>, Operation CASTLE (1954)
Dated: 8 December 1993

RAEM/NTPR
8 December 1993

Memorandum For Record

Radiation Dose Assessment for Operation CASTLE (1954)

Purpose

This memorandum assesses the dose from external emitters, and from internally deposited radionuclides, that was accrued by the subject named veteran during his participation in atmospheric nuclear weapon testing.

Background

Operation CASTLE was the series of nuclear weapon tests conducted at the Pacific Proving Ground (PPG) in 1954. The PPG, located in the Central Pacific Ocean area, consists of the land areas, lagoons, and waters within 3 miles of two Marshall Islands Atolls, Enewetak and Bikini. Bikini Atoll is about 2200 nautical miles southwest of Hawaii, and Enewetak Atoll is about 195 nautical miles west of Bikini Atoll. Enewetak Atoll and Bikini Atoll consist of 35 and 26 islands, respectively, and each Atoll has a total land area of about 2.7 square miles. The principal objective of Operation CASTLE was to test high-yield thermonuclear devices. (Reference 1).

Table 1 presents shot data on the nuclear shots fired during CASTLE. All CASTLE shots were fired at Bikini Atoll except for NECTAR, which was fired at Enewetak Atoll. Note that MT is the acronym for "megaton." (References 1 & 2)

Table 1. Operation CASTLE nuclear shot data.

Shot	1954 Date	Time	Type	Yield (MT)
BRAVO	1 March	0645	surface	15
ROMEO	27 March	0630	barge	11
KOON	7 April	0620	surface	0.11
UNION	26 April	0605	barge	6.9
YANKEE	5 May	0610	barge	13.5
NECTAR	14 May	0620	barge	1.69

The veteran was transferred from USS BELLE GROVE (LSD 2) to LST-762 [later christened USS FLOYD COUNTY (LST 762)] on 21 January. (Unless otherwise stated, all dates in this assessment are in 1954.) During CASTLE, the veteran was an Electronics Technician Third Class, U.S. Navy, in LST-762 (Reference 3). Personnel in that rating maintain and repair shipboard electronic equipment (Reference 4). The veteran was on duty in LST-762 until 29 February 1956 (Reference 3).

During CASTLE, LST-762 was assigned to Task Unit 7.3.9, Transport Unit. As part of TU 7.3.9, LST-762 transported shot devices, passengers, and freight between Enewetak Atoll and Bikini Atoll (Reference 1). The earliest known date of LST-762's arrival at PPG in conjunction with CASTLE is 20 October 1953. According to the ship's deck log, LST-762 departed PPG on 27 April enroute to Pearl Harbor. (Reference 3)

Film Badge Dosimetry

Radiological safety records for personnel in LST-762 include "cohort" film badges for the period 10 to 16 March, individual film badges for one-day periods, and medical record entries. Cohort badge #8787 was issued to one sailor, and that reading was used as a dose of record for eleven LST-762 personnel, including the veteran, for 10 to 16 March. Three individual film badges were issued to the veteran. Data on each of his film badges are presented in Table 2. (References 1 & 5)

#1

In accordance with provisions set forth in Reference 6, the film badge return dates, which were not documented, are inferred; and doses entered into medical records for LST-762 personnel, which were intended to cover unbadged periods, are disregarded in lieu of reconstructed doses for those periods.

Table 2. Film badge data.

Film Badge #	Issue Date	Return Date	Process Date	Reading (R)	
8787	10 March	16 March	n/a	0.335	Cohort Badge
14903	31 March	31 March	n/a	0.500	Individual Badges
14104	1 April	1 April	n/a	0.245	
14118	4 April	4 April	n/a	0.410	

For the limited badge periods shown in Table 2 and given the known radiation environment in LST-762, the film badge readings are high. This analysis regards the data in Table 2 as true, and the film badge reading "excess" will be used to high-side the calculation of the veteran's internal dose.

#2

Radiation Environment (Reference 5)

The peak fallout intensities in LST-762 during CASTLE are shown in Table 3.

Residual contamination in Bikini Lagoon from BRAVO contributal to the accrual of dose by personnel in LST-762. Contaminants produced ambient intensity over the surface of the lagoon, adhered to the ship's hull, and were circulated in the ship's sea water systems.

Because of mechanical difficulties, the ship was unable to make good speed in its passage to Pearl Harbor, and on 5 May was taken in tow by LST-975. YANKEE fallout descended on LST-762 on 6 May, more than one week after the ship departed PPG.

Table 3. Peak fallout intensities, LST-762.

Shot	mR/hour	H + hours
BRAVO	10	16
ROMEO	8.5	77.5
YANKEE	39.7	35.3

Assumptions & Exposure Scenario

The veteran is assumed to have participated in the activities listed below, which resulted in his potential accrual of dose from CASTLE residual contamination.

- He was in LST-762 during that ship's tour of duty in PPG from 19 January to 27 April, and he remained a member of the ship's crew through 29 February 1956.
- He was a generic crew member in LST-762.

Dose From Initial Radiation (References 5 & 7)

Personnel in LST-762 were too distant from any CASTLE shot to have accrued from them a measurable initial neutron or gamma radiation dose.

Dose From External Emitters (Reference 5)

The reconstructed external gamma dose from fallout for generic personnel who were topside 40%—and below decks 60%—of the time from 1 March to 25 July, when the dose rate fell to less than 0.001 rem per day, is 1.068 rem. Because the veteran's film badge readings cover part of that period, reconstructed doses will be applied only for the unbadged periods. Table 4 provides details about the veteran's gamma (γ) dose from his participation in CASTLE.

Dose From Internal Emitters (References 5, 8, & 9)

In calculating the veteran's (50-year) committed dose equivalent to the kidneys from internally deposited radionuclides, the following scenarios and potential pathways were considered:

- He inhaled descending BRAVO, ROMEO, and YANKEE fallout throughout each period of deposition.
- He inhaled resuspended fallout in LST-762 for 100 hours after cessation of deposition.

Because LST-762 employed its washdown system only after the descent on the ship of YANKEE fallout, this assessment assumes that the BRAVO and ROMEO fallout that was resuspended by walking on weather decks or in enclosed spaces in LST-762 is characterized by a resuspension factor of $10^{-5}m^{-1}$. In this case, the appropriate resuspension factor for YANKEE fallout is $10^{-6}m^{-1}$. The veteran's breathing rate throughout periods of inhalation of descending and resuspended fallout is assumed to have been 1.2 m^3 hr^{-1}.

As stated above, the veteran's film badge readings are higher than the reconstructed doses for personnel in LST-762 for the same periods. To high-side the calculation of his internal dose, the “excess” film badge reading is assumed to have been accrued concurrently with his inhalation of resuspended fallout. Table 4 presents the fallout sources and “excess” doses for each film badge.

#3

Film Badge Number	“Excess” Reading (R)	Fallout Source
8787	0.287	BRAVO
14903	0.454	ROMEO
14104	0.211	ROMEO
14118	0.392	ROMEO

The veteran's (50-year) committed dose equivalent to the kidneys from inhaling descending and resuspended fallout, as described above, is 0.028 rem.

#4

External Dose & Participation Summary

Based on the foregoing facts aad assumptions, the veteran's gamma (γ) dose by date period for his participation in Operation CASTLE is presented in Table 5. His neutron dose for CASTLE is zero rem.

Table 5. External dose and participation summary.

Dates (yymmdd)	γ Dose (rem)	Remark
540119 - 540228	0	No Exposure Potential
540301 - 540309	0.198	Reconstruction
540310 - 540316	0.335	Film Badge
540317 - 540330	0.135	Reconstruction
540331	0.500	Film Badge
540401	0.245	Film Badge
54540402 - 540403	0.048	Reconstruction
540404	0.410	Film Badge
540405 - 540703	0.516	Reconstruction
Total =	2.4	Upper Bound = 3.5 rem

Internal (kidney,) Dose Summary 50-year committed dose equivalent: <0.15 rem.

References

1. "CASTLE Series – 1954," DNA 6035F , 1 April 1982 .
2. "Announced United States Nuclear Tests. July 1945 Through December 1992." DOE/NV—209 (Rev. 13) , May 1993 .
3. Documents located in the veteran's NTPR file .
4. "The Bluejacket's Manual," Fourteenth Edition , U.S. Naval Institute , 1950 .
5. "Analysis of Radiation Exposure For Naval Personnel at Operation CASTLE," DNA-TR-84-6 , 28 February 1984 .
6. "Operation CASTLE Dosimetry Purification Procedures, Revision 1," Reynolds Electrical & Engineering Co., Inc. , May 1993 .
7. "Neutron Exposure For DOD Nuclear Test Personnel," DNA-TR-84-405 , 15 August 1985 .
8. "FIIDOS—A Computer Code For the Computation of Fallout Inhalation and Ingestion to Organs," DNA-TR-84-375 , 12 December 1985 .
9. Shot-specific radiochemical data .

H

Example of Traceability of Dose Data

Appendix H-1 is a printout (4 pages) from the database for an individual who participated in the BUSTER-JANGLE, CASTLE, CROSSROADS and UPSHOT-KNOTHOLE test series. For BUSTER-JANGLE, this individual participated from November 26 through December 1, 1951. Entries for individual days (H-1 #1) indicate the dose (H-1 #2), the type of dosimetry device [H-1 #3], and the badge number (H-1 #4).

The lack of entries in the last column (H-1 #5) indicated that these are initial entries with no subsequent changes. This individual also participated in the CASTLE series (H-1, #6) from February 11 through May 14, 1954, with a personal badge worn for ten periods and a cohort badge reading assigned for March 11 (H-1 #7).

All of these entries, which account for 1,270 mrem, were either newly entered or changed on 29 March 1994 (H-1 #8), following the dose reconstruction dated 27 February 1994 (Appendix H-2). From the database, it is not possible to know what dose information was contained in the computer record prior to this recent dose reconstruction; that is, were badge data for CASTLE included and, if so, why were they changed?

This individual was not badged during four time intervals for which reconstructed doses are shown (H-1 #9). The database indicates that this individual participated in the UPSHOT-KNOTHOLE series from 30 March through 5 June 1953 (H-l #10). Personal film badges were issued for 11 intervals (H-1 #11), but several intervals are not included, including 1 April through 11 May, which is not fully covered in the dose reconstruction document (Appendix H-2).

H-1

Personal Information Form — Dose Assignment, NTPR Database

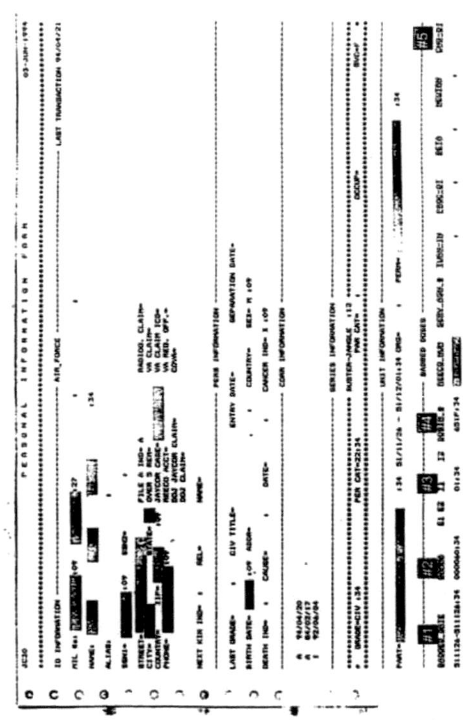

Appendix H-1, Personal Information Form - Dose Assignment, NTPR Database, Page 1

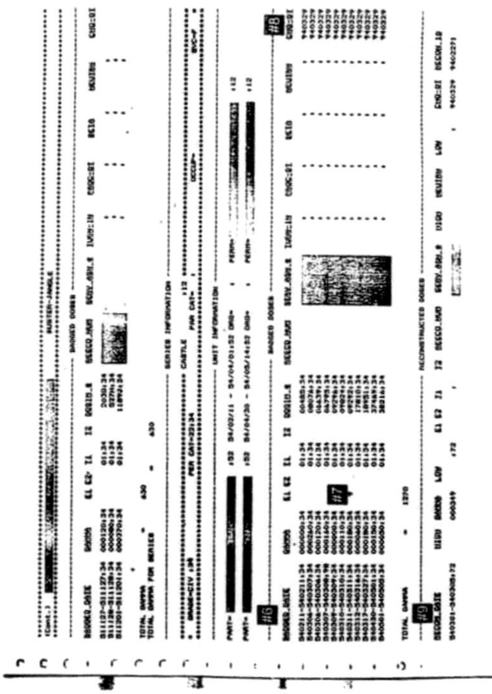

Appendix H-1, Personal Information Form - Dose Assignment, NTPR Database, Page 2

(Cont.) [redacted] CASTLE

RECONSTRUCTED DOSES

RECON_DATE	HIGH	GAMMA	LOW	E1 E2	I1	I2	REECO_NUM	SERV_ABN_#	HIGH	NEUTRN	LOW	CHG:DT	RECON_ID
540309-540311:72		000049	:72		:						:	940329	9402271
540328-540331:72		000509	:72		:						:	940329	9402271
540506-540514:72		000034	:73		:						:	940329	9402271

TOTAL GAMMA = 941
TOTAL GAMMA FOR SERIES = 2211

SERIES INFORMATION

CROSSROADS :10
GRADE=BN :29 PER CAT=04:07 PAR CAT= : OCCUP= SVC=N

UNIT INFORMATION

PART= [redacted] :27 46/07/01 - 46/12/07:15 ORG= : PERM=

RECONSTRUCTED DOSES

RECON_DATE	HIGH	GAMMA	LOW	E1 E2	I1	I2	REECO_NUM	SERV_ABN_#	HIGH	NEUTRN	LOW	CHG:DT	RECON_ID
460701-461207:72		000723	:72		:		[redacted]				:		9402271

TOTAL GAMMA = 723
TOTAL GAMMA FOR SERIES = 723

SERIES INFORMATION

POSTUPKN :34
GRADE= : PER CAT=22:34 PAR CAT= : OCCUP= SVC=F

UNIT INFORMATION

PART= [redacted] :34 53/11/02 - 54/11/05:34 ORG= : PERM= [redacted] :34

BADGED DOSES

BADGED_DATE	GAMMA	E1 E2	I1	I2	DOSID_#	REECO_NUM	SERV_ABN_#	IVNV:IN	PROC:DT	BETA	NEUTRN	CHG:DT
531103-531103:34	000020:34		01:34		018329:34	[redacted]		:	:	:	:	

Appendix H-1, Personal Information Form - Dose Assignment, NTPR Database, Page 3

```
*****************************************************************************************
(Cont.) [redacted]                         POSTUPKN
*****************************************************************************************

------------------------------------ BADGED DOSES ---------------------------------------
BADGED_DATE           GAMMA     E1 E2  I1    I2  DOSIM_#    RECCO_NUM  SERV_ASN_#  TUBS:IN  PROC:DT  BETA  NEUTRN  CHG:DT
531104-531104:34   000040:34           01:34    018014:34  [redacted]

TOTAL GAMMA               =      40
TOTAL GAMMA FOR SERIES             =     40

----------------------------------- SERIES INFORMATION ----------------------------------
************************************************* UPSHOT-KNOTHOLE:34 ********************
*  GRADE=CIV :34           PER CAT=22:34                 PAR CAT=   :          OCCUP=          SVC=F  *
*****************************************************************************************
----------------------------- #10 ---- UNIT INFORMATION ---------------------------------
PART=[redacted]  :34  53/03/30 - 53/04/05:15 ORG=   :   PERM=[redacted]  :12

-- #11 ------------------------------------ BADGED DOSES --------------------------------
BADGED_DATE           GAMMA     E1 E2  I1    I2  DOSIM_#    RECCO_NUM  SERV_ASN_#  TUBS:IN  PROC:DT  BETA  NEUTRN  CHG:DT
530331-530331:34   000020:34           01:34    000017:34  [redacted]
530312-530312:34   000240:34           01:34    014218:34
530313-530313:34   000000:34           01:34    012646:34
530314-530314:34   000250:34           01:34    029310:34
530315-530315:34   000190:34           01:34    013805:34
530316-530316:34   000130:34           01:34    013693:34
530318-530318:34   000130:34           01:34    012640:34
530325-530325:34   000020:34           01:34    015985:34
530327-530327:34   000130:34           01:34    016173:34
530329-530329:34   000000:34           01:34    016853:34
530401-530401:34   000250:34           01:34    017070:34

TOTAL GAMMA               =      1370
TOTAL GAMMA FOR SERIES             =     1370

TOTAL ALL GAMMA                    =     4994
```

Appendix H-1, Personal Information Form - Dose Assignment, NTPR Database, Page 4

H-2

Memorandum from SAIC to DNA-RAEM/NTPR

Subject: Dose Reconstruction: <NAME> Operation CROSSROADS (1946), BUSTER-JANGLE, (1951), UPSHOT-KNOTHOLE (1953), CASTLE (1954)
Date: 27 February 1994

DNA-RAEM/NTPR (M. Owais)

Memorandum For Record

Dose Reconstruction for_________

Operations CROSSROADS (1946), BUSTER-JANGLE (1951), UPSHOT-KNOTHOLE (1953), CASTLE (1954)

Introduction:

At the time of Operation CROSSROADS, (then) Motor Machinist's Mate 2nd Class___was a crew member on the USS SYLVANIA (AKA 44). The Standard Engineering Dose applies, and is available from the data in References 9 and 10. During BUSTER-JANGLE, UPSHOT-KNOTHOLE, and CASTLE, the veteran was a civilian working for For B-J and U-K, film badge data is available for all periods during which the veteran would have been exposed. For CASTLE, some film badge data is available, and dose reconstruction is used here for the remainder of the time.

Operation CROSSROADS:

The veteran was a Motor Machinist's Mate 2nd Class aboard the SYLVANIA, and is assigned the Standard Engineering Dose. From the methodology and data contained in References 9 and 10, for the SYLVANIA this dose is 0.723 rem.

Operation BUSTER-JANGLE:

During Operation BUSTER-JANGLE, the veteran was a civilian working for

Film badge data for the veteran are available for the dates 26, 27, 28 November, and 1 December 1951. References 11, 12, and 13 show that : was only involved at Shot UNCLE. Reference 14 indicates that personnel were not allowed into the display area before 1 Dec 1951, two days after the detonation. Thus, it would appear that the available film badge data covers all times that the veteran might have been exposed to radiation during Operation BUSTER-JANGLE. The first three film badge dates are for equipment set-up prior to Shot UNCLE. The reason that there was non-zero exposure is that the UNCLE display area lay in the fallout field of the previous shot, Shot SUGAR. The cumulative total of the four badge readings is 0.630 rem.

Operation UPSHOT-KNOTHOLE:

During Operation UPSHOT-KNOTHOLE, the veteran was a civilian working for

Film badge data for the veteran are available for the dates 31 March and 12, 13, 14, 15, 16, 18, 25, 27, 29 May and 1 June 1953. Experience has shown that the UPSHOT-KNOTHOLE film badge data is reasonably complete, and that the film badge records of any one individual usually covers the entire dose that the individual received during the whole of UPSHOT-KNOTHOLE. After examining the veteran film badge records, along with those of the other personnel involved with UPSHOT-KNOTHOLE, it appears that those badges dated 1 June were actually worn during the recovery operations following Shot CLIMAX on 4 June. Among the personnel film badge records, there is no record dated 4 June, when substantial recovery activity took place following the CLIMAX detonation. All personnel, on the other hand, have records date 1 June, and all are in the range 255 to 285 mR. Reconstruction shows this to be about what they would have received on 4 June, and there is no possibility of anyone receiving this dose on 1 June. The total film badge dose of the veteran for U-K is 1.370 rem. the veteran accrued an additional 0.060 rem in November 1953.

Operation CASTLE:

The attached table summarizes the locations and doses used for the veteran dose reconstruction. There are film-badge records for the veteran for most of the period in question. For the remainder of the time, the use of the Reference 3 information and reasonable assumptions is considered to lead to reliable results. For instance, Reference 3 could not establish whether or not the veteran remained on the USNS AINSWORTH (TAP 181) during the period of March 2 - 4, when the ship was anchored at Enewetak Atoll. Since the veteran was a civilian, not a crew member, one might normally assume that he and the other civilians spent those days ashore at Enewetak. Radiation safety is an additional consideration in support of this assumption. Comparing Reference 5, pages 80 and 119 shows that the radiation intensity aboard the AINSWORTH was higher than that on Enewetak by roughly a factor of 3 or so. Thus, the assumption that the civilians stayed ashore during this period is reasonable.

Reference 3 shows the AINSWORTH arriving at Bikini Atoll at 0900 on 5 Mar 54. Reference 6 lists one boat mission (LCU #638) with Project 3.2 people for that date, but the names listed do not include the veteran. The radiation levels at Bikini locations Nan and Tare for that day average about 1 and 0.15 R/hr, respectively (Reference 7, p.76). These intensities are much higher that the intensity on the AINSWORTH (Reference 5, p.80), so that rad-safe considerations would have dictated that personnel stay aboard ship except at times when necessary duties dictated otherwise. Thus, when neither film badge records nor any other indication of the veteran' presence elsewhere can be found, it is assumed that he remained aboard ship at Bikini. Reference 6 shows him on a helicopter on March 7, a day for which a film-badge reading is available. For March 11, Reference 6 shows the veteran and [coworker] on a helicopter mission. There is no badge reading available for the veteran for that day, but there is one for [coworker] (Reference 3). Therefore, [coworker]'s badge reading is used.

Reference 3 has the pre-KOON and pre-UNION surveys taking place prior to 1 April. In case these activities did not fall on days covered by the veteran' known film badge records, a separate day for each pre-shot survey was assumed. The fallout field plot in Reference 7, p. 99, was used as a basis for determining the radiation intensity to which the veteran was exposed. A time of about 2 hours was assumed for the time duration of each survey.

The period of May 6 - 14 is without documentation. The assumption that the veteran spent this time at Enewetak is not critical, since he would have received about the same dose had he remained aboard the AINSWORTH.

Page 3

Dose Summary:

Neutron : < 0.001 rem

Gamma :

Time period	Dose(rem)	Method
01 Jul 46 - 07 Dec 46	0.723	Reconstruction
26 Nov 51 - 26 Nov 51	0.060	Film Badge (651 F)
27 Nov 51 - 27 Nov 51	0.120	Film Badge (203 G)
28 Nov 51 - 28 Nov 51	0.080	Film Badge (527 H)
01 Dec 51 - 01 Dec 51	0.370	Film Badge (1189 J)
31 Mar 53 - 31 Mar 53	0.020	Film Badge (000017)
12 May 53 - 12 May 53	0.240	Film Badge (014318)
13 May 53 - 13 May 53	0.000	Film Badge (012646)
14 May 53 - 14 May 53	0.255	Film Badge (029310)
15 May 53 - 15 May 53	0.190	Film Badge (013805)
16 May 53 - 16 May 53	0.130	Film Badge (013693)
18 May 53 - 18 May 53	0.130	Film Badge (012668)
25 May 53 - 25 May 53	0.020	Film Badge (015985)
27 May 53 - 27 May 53	0.130	Film Badge (016173)
29 May 53 - 29 May 53	0.000	Film Badge (016853)
01 Jun 53 - 01 Jun 53	0.255	Film Badge (017070)
03 Nov 53 - 03 Nov 53	0.020	Film Badge (018329)
04 Nov 53 - 04 Nov 53	0.040	Film Badge (018014)
11 Feb 54 - 11 Feb 54	0.000	Film Badge (00485)
01 Mar 54 - 05 Mar 54	0.349	Reconstruction
06 Mar 54 - 06 Mar 54	0.120	Film Badge (06639)
06 Mar 54 - 07 Mar 54	0.260	Film Badge (08076)
07 Mar 54 - 08 Mar 54 (est.)	0.160	Film Badge (06795)
09 Mar 54 - 09 Mar 54	0.000	Film Badge (09296)
09 Mar 54 - 11 Mar 54	0.049	Reconstruction
10 Mar 54 - 10 Mar 54	0.110	Film Badge (09824)
11 Mar 54 - 11 Mar 54	0.180	Film Badge (09292)(with [coworker])
12 Mar 54 - 16 Mar 54	0.060	Film Badge (17810)
17 Mar 54 - 27 Mar 54	0.180	Film Badge (18951)
28 Mar 54 - 31 Mar 54	0.509	Reconstruction
30 Apr 54 - 01 May 54	0.150	Film Badge (37469)
01 May 54 - 05 May 54	0.050	Film Badge (38216)
06 May 54 - 14 May 54	0.034	Reconstruction
Total =	5.0 rem (upper bound 6.7)	

References

1. Memorandum: “Dose Reconstruction,___,” I. Kesselman , JAYCOR , 06 July 1993 .
2. NUCLEAR TEST PERSONNEL REVIEW , Telephone Information Form,___, 27 January 92 .
3. “Chronology of the Veteran's Movements,” unsigned but apparently from JAYCOR , 16 July 92 .
4. “Operation CASTLE, Project 3.2, Crater Survey,” HQ Field Command, AFSWC, Sandia Base , Albuquerque NM , WT-920 (EX) , June 1955 .

5. "Analysis of Radiation Exposure for Naval Personnel at Operation CASTLE," DNA-TR-84-6 , Defense Nuclear Agency , 28 February 1984 .
6. "Bikini Daily Diaries," Operation CASTLE , 1 March 1954 - 14 May 1954 .
7. "Distribution and Intensity of Fallout," Project 2.5a, Operation CASTLE , R.L. Steton , et al , WT-915 , January 1956 .
8. Letter to the veteran, 981T3FD/2008, from W. H. Loeffler, Captain USN, Navy Nuclear Test Personnel Review, 17 February 1984 .
9. "Analysis of Radiation Exposure for Naval Units of Operation Crossroads, Volume I Basic Report," DNA-TR-82-05-V1 , Defense Nuclear Agency , 3 March 1982 .
10. "Analysis of Radiation Exposure for Naval Units of Operation Crossroads, Volume III (Appendix B), Support Ships," DNA-TR-82-05-V3 , Defense Nuclear Agency , 3 March 1982 .
11. "Operation BUSTER-JANGLE, 1951," Defense Nuclear Agency , DNA 6023F , 21 June 1982 .
12. "Shots ABLE to EASY, The First Five Shots of the BUSTER-JANGLE Series," DNA 6024F , Defense Nuclear Agency , 22 June 1982 .
13. "Shots SUGAR and UNCLE, The Final Tests of the BUSTER-JANGLE Series," DNA 6025F , Defense Nuclear Agency , 23 June 1982 .
14. "Analysis of Radiation Exposure for Military Participants, Exercises Desert Rock I, II, & III, Operation BUSTER-JANGLE," DNA-TR-87-116 , Defense Nuclear Agency , 22 December 1987 .
15. "Analysis of Radiation Exposure for Troop Observers, Exercise Desert Rock V, Operation UPSHOT-KNOTHOLE," DNA 5742F , Defense Nuclear Agency , 28 April 1981 .
16. "Operation UPSHOT-KNOTHOLE, 1953," DNA 6014F , 11 January 1982 .
17. "Shots ANNIE to RAY, The First Five Tests of the UPSHOT-KNOTHOLE Series, 17 March - 11 April 1953," DNA 6017F , 14 January 1982 .
18. "Shot BADGER, A Test of the UPSHOT-KNOTHOLE Series, 18 April 1953," DNA 6015F , 12 January 1982 .
19. "Shot SIMON, A Test of the UPSHOT-KNOTHOLE Series, 25 April 1953," DNA 6016F , 13 January 1982 .
20. "Shots ENCORE to CLIMAX, The Final Four Tests of the UPSHOT-KNOTHOLE Series, 8 May - 4 June 1953," DNA 6018F , 15 January 1982 .
21. "Operation UPSHOT-KNOTHOLE, Radiological Safety Operation," Tom. D. Collison , AFSWP , WT-702 (REF.) , June 1953 .

SUMMARY OF VETERAN'S RADIATION DOSE OPERATION CASTLE

			REFERENCES	
DATE	LOCATION	DOSE (mrem)	DOSES	LOCATION
March 01	AINSWORTH	125 *	Ref.5,p.134	Ref.3
March 02-04	Enewetak	161	Ref.5,p.119	Ref.3; see text
March 05	AINSWORTH	63	Ref.5,p.134	Ref.3; see text
March 06		120	BADGE (06639)	
March 06-07	surveyed BRAVO crater	260	BADGE (08076)	Ref.4
March 07-08		160	BADGE (06795)	
March 09		0	BADGE (09296)	
March 09-11	AINSWORTH	49	Ref.5,p.134	Ref.3; see text
March 10		110	BADGE (09824)	
March 11	helicopter	180	BADGE (09292, [coworker])	
March 12-16		60	BADGE (17810)	
March 17-27		180	BADGE (18951)	
March 28-31	AINSWORTH	469	Ref.5,p.134	Ref.3; see text
March 29	pre-KOON survey	Ref.7,p.99	30	Ref.3; Ref. 4
March 30	pre-UNION survey	10	Ref.7,p.99	Ref.3; Ref. 4
April 01-29	returned to ZI	0	Ref.3	
April 30-May 01		150	BADGE (37469)	
May 01-05		50	BADGE (38216)	
May 06-14	Enewetak	34	Ref.5,p.119	see text
	TOTAL DOSE =	2211 mrem		

* Reconstructed dose was used in lieu of assessed dose for 01 March

I

Potential for Bias due to Differential Methods of Dose Assignment

Comparison of Doses Assigned to Atomic Test Participants Who Had Individual Dose Reconstructions and Those Who Did Not

The Dosimetry Working Group of the Committee to Study the Mortality of Military Personnel Present at Atmospheric Tests of Nuclear Weapons (Five-Series Study) attempted to quantify the effect of differences in dose assignment methodologies between those who had an individual dose reconstruction and those who did not. It is impossible to do this directly, since exact individual doses are unknown. Adopting an indirect approach, the Working Group first assembled dose data on Five-Series participants who had individualized reconstructions.

The Working Group used, as a benchmark, the doses that had been entered for these individuals in the original Five-Series Study (NRC 1985). Because these benchmark doses could have a tendency to increase or decrease over time within the Five-Series cohort as a whole, a comparison group was also assembled. Changes in dose assignments for the comparison group presumably reflect the updating and cleaning activities that have been carried out by the DNA and its contractors since the creation of the 1985 NRC analysis file.

The Working Group identified 277 participants (members of the Five-Series cohort) who:

- had a dose in the 1985 data file,
- had been referred to SAIC for dosimetry, and
- could be matched to a person in the current (May 1994) data file.

For comparison, the Working Group randomly selected 415 participants who had an entry in both 1985 and current data files, but whose dose had not been referred for individualized reconstruction. In this set of individualized reconstructions and controls, a number of individuals were found to have missing dose values. Those individuals were eliminated from further consideration, leaving 195 individualized reconstruction cases and 269 nonindividualized reconstruction cases.

To be included in this comparison, an individual had to have nonmissing external gamma dose data for each of the five test series in which he participated. These nonmissing components were summed to give a total gamma dose. Doses from tests other than those included in the Five-Series Study were not considered, because those data were not available in the 1985 data set.

The differences between the paired dose entries (1985 data matched to the current data) are summarized in Table 2. The currently assigned doses tend to be higher than their 1985 counterparts, and the tendency is highly statistically significant within each group ($p < .0001$, sign test). Also, the pattern of the changes is different between the individualized vs. nonindividualized doses, that is the two categorized distributions of paired differences are dissimilar ($x^2(3) > 70$, $p < .0001$).

Despite the highly significant difference between the dose changes experienced by the individualized vs. nonindividualized groups, one can see that the primary source of the discrepancy is the relatively greater tendency for the nonindividualized dose estimates to stay the same. If one repeats the comparison, removing participants whose doses stayed the same, there is no difference at all ($x^2(2) = 1.9$, $p > .3$) in the pattern of the changes. Thus, these data suggest that when the dose was changed by the individualized reconstruction methods, there was *not* a tendency for the change to be greater or less than that for a participant whose dose also changed because of alterations in the unit-based assignments.

Table 2. Numbers of Participants Categorized by the Difference, $\Delta D = (Dc-Do)$, Between Their Current Dose (Dc) and Original Dose Assigned in 1985 (Do) for Each Dose Assignment Method (individualized and nonindividualized)

Dose Assignment Method	Dose Decreased, $\Delta D < 0$ mrem	No Change, $\Delta D = 0$ mrem	Dose Increased, $0 < \Delta D < 1{,}001$ mrem	Dose Increased, $\Delta D > 1{,}000$ mrem
Individually reconstructed	12 (6 %)	60 (31 %)	88 (45 %)	35 (18 %)
Not individually reconstructed	7 (3 %)	191 (71 %)	44 (16 %)	27 (10 %)

This evaluation was not an exhaustive study of potential biases in the NTPR dose database. In fact, there are several notable caveats to consider. First, the NTPR database is constantly being updated. This study used dose data from the Five-Series Study frozen at two moments in time, separated by about 10 years. Clean up of the current dose data for the Five-Series Study is still in progress and will not be completed until 1996.

The results presented here should not be interpreted as a demonstration that there are no systematic differences between individualized and nonindividualized dose assignments. We do not know the true dose for any participant, and thus have no direct menus to assess bias. Moreover, participants were to some extent self-selected to have an individualized reconstruction, and their real doses may be higher or lower on average than those for the remainder of the cohort. Also, doses assigned to the same participants for series other than the five might have revealed a very different pattern, as the dose data for other series have not been cleaned as completely. These other series doses would be relevant to computing a total gamma dose for analysis of potential health effects.

The process of generating these data revealed some perplexing results for individuals in the database. These included significant differences between assigned doses in the current (May 1994) data file and corresponding SAIC dose reconstructions. There were numerous instances in which the database does not seem to reflect SAIC reconstructions completed several years ago. In some cases, the current dose data are missing despite the existence of individualized reconstructions. As noted above, these could be the result of the incomplete cleanup of the dose values in the current data set or there may be other reasons for the disparities.

The Working Group attempted to quantify possible bias in the Five-Series dose data that could have resulted from different treatment of those who had individualized reconstructions and those who did not. This was done by comparing the dose entered in the data file for the 1985 Five Series Study (NRC, 1985b) with that in the current data file, for all participants whose name had been referred to SAIC for an individualized dose reconstruction and for a comparison group of participants who had not had an individualized reconstruction. Participants with individualized reconstructions were more likely than those without individualized reconstructions to have had their doses modified between 1985 and 1994. In both groups, when there was a change in the assigned dose, it was much more likely to be an increase than a decrease.

When individuals whose doses did not change over time were eliminated from consideration, no differences were found in the pattern of changes in dose between the individualized and nonindividualized groups. That is, between these two groups, no difference was detected in the proportion of participants who fell into categories defined by whether their doses went down, went up by a little (up to 1 rem), or went up by a lot (more than 1 rem). Thus, for those individuals whose dose *did* change, it did not appear to make a difference whether they received an individual reconstruction or not. This suggests that the individualized dose reconstruction methodology was not systematically biased relative to the generic "cleaning" of the data.

These findings do not, however, allay one of the Working Group's most serious concerns over differential dose assignment — that individualized doses could have experienced a significantly different pattern of change than nonindividualized doses. For those individuals whose doses did change, it did not appear to make a difference whether they received an individual reconstruction or not. Nevertheless, the patterns of change shown in the above table of differences (Table 2) do suggest that those with individualized reconstructions will tend to have higher assigned doses than those without individualized reconstructions. This could bias any dose-response analysis based on the existing data.

APPENDIX B

National Association of Atomic Veterans Medical Survey

"NAAV Data Center" **2310 Apollo Way, Mesquite, Texas 75150-5329** FAX: 214/216-1838

March 9, 1995

J.C. Johnson,
Ph.D., CHP
National Academy of Sciences Institute of Medicine, Medical Follow-Up Agency 2101 Constitution Avenue Washington, D.C. 20418

Dear Dr. Johnson,

In reply to your letter of March 7, 1995, requesting registration criteria utilized to select Atomic Veterans to be placed on the NAAV Registry, the following is submitted for your information.

Since the formation of NAAV in 1978, various personnel have attempted to compile data an the medical problems faced by veterans who participated during the period of "Atmosphere Testing". Additionally, those veterans who were POW's and those veterans who were occupation troops near Hiroshima and Nagasaki have been included with the test personnel. Together these veterans have come to be known as "Atomic Veterans".

During my tenure as the National Commander and NAAV Board Chairman from 1986 through 1989, I discovered records and files of various Medical Surveys which had been conducted by NAAV. in 1992, we started collecting these survey forms in one file location, cataloging them by Test Series, and entering the data from these survey forms into a computer data base (FileMaker II and then FileMaker Pro) where the various categories of information are sortable into desired and usable data. Our present Medical Survey Questionnaire was developed at that time. Each new member since mid 1992 has been requested to complete a survey form for our records. Presently, I receive an average about 10 of these survey forms each week.

The following sources of information are utilized to compile information on each veteran listed in the NAAV Medical Survey Data Registry:

a. A NAAV Medical Survey Questionnaire completed by the veteran or his widow. Specifically the years 1980, 1983, 1985-1986, 1992-1995. Many questionnaires are accompanied by copies of orders, DD-214 forms, discharge papers, doctors and hospital reports, VA documents, and DNA correspondence and/or registry forms.

b. Correspondence files containing letters of inquires from veterans, their widows or children along with discharge documents, copies of orders, media articles, Guinea Pig Certificates, Letters of Commendation, VA documents and claim forms, etc.

c. Information furnished by widows, ie, Death Certificates, DD-214 Forms, discharge papers, newspaper articles, VA documents and claim forms, etc.

All of this information is being sorted, cataloged, and entered into the NAAV computer data base to provide NAAV management with facts and figures usable in our efforts to "Obtain Simple Justice".

In addition to Test Personnel, we are collecting Medical Survey information on other classes of exposed veterans. What could be termed the second generation Atomic Veteran. Personnel involved in Broken Arrow incidents, nuclear submarine crewmen, nuclear weapons handlers and custodians, etc. I have about 150 of this category so far.

We don't usually hear from a veteran until he connects in his mind that his health problems might be related to his exposure. Also widows discover who we are and contact us concerning their husbands involvement in nuclear testing. Since we operate on members dues and member donations only, we have little money to advertise the plight of atomic veterans and their families and even less to utilize on a project such as this registry. This registry is my labor of love for the last three years with a little help from my friends. If any of you fat cats have any grant money laying around, I could put it to good use for stationary supplies, postage, data entry, and phone bills.

The data furnished you recently is but a snap shot of our registry. By the end of this year we hope to have available on the NAAV Registry most of the health survey information collected by NAAV on Atomic Veterans over the past 18 years. At that point we will add Correspondence file and data received from Widows to the registry.

Unfortunately, much information has been lost because of veteran deaths and by a government who covered up individual's stupidity because they put security before compassion, fear of lawsuits above individual suffering, and official's pride and ego over truth.

I am personally very pleased that the data transfer was successful. I regret that not all of the information on Crossroad veterans is completed as I still have to enter information on personnel from the Radiological Safety Section and the Ammunition Disposal Teams during Operation Crossroads. Perhaps you will accept and update sometime in the future.

I hope that some time in the future I might be able to study your report and conclusions. Please feel free to call on me for any assistance I might be able to furnish the Crossroads study or the Five Tests study.

I remain,

Sincerely,

Boley H. Caldwell III
LTC(Ret)
U.S. Army

NATIONAL ASSOCIATION
OF
ATOMIC VETERANS

Medical History & Data Questionnaire

When Completed, Please Return to
NAAV, P.O. BOX 4424
SALEM, MA 01970

From time to time it is necessary for NAAV to provide statistical medical information on Atomic Veterans to our members, the news media, to Congress in support of legislation, the Department of Veterans' Affairs, the Department of Justice, and other government agencies. Without having a readily available medical data base on you, your children and grandchildren, we can not properly represent you.The last up date of our data files was in 1986, therefore we are requesting Atomic Veterans to complete this questionnaire and return it to NAAV as soon as possible.

If the individual veteran is deceased, it is particularly important that this questionnaire be completed as accurately as possible by a relative or friend. If possible, please enclose a copy of the Death Certificate with this completed questionnaire.

No information released will be in violation of the "Privacy Act". For the most part the information released is in the form of statistics. Most questions are straight forward but if you have a question please do not hesitate to contact us.

IMPORTANT: Please read the following statement, sign and date on the lines provided. Your signature is required. Thank you.

I understand that this information is needed so that NAAV can help with problems that I may have and so that certain medical research authorities, with NAAV's approval, may pursue medical problems of importance to all Atomic Veterans. The information I provide may be used by NAAV to advance the cause of the Atomic Veterans.

____
(Signature)

____
(Date)

PART I: Personal Information

1. Your Name - as spelled while in the military (or as a civilian employee).
First: ____________ Middle: ____________ Last: ____________
2. Your address where you can be contacted
Address: ______________________________
City: ____________ State: ________ ZIP Code: ________
3. Telephone Number: (Include Area Code) (____) ____ - ______
4. Birth Date: Month ____ Day ____ Year ____
5. Sex: Male _ Female _ Race: ______ 6. SSN: ___ - __ - ____
7. Branch of Service: ______ 8. Military Service No: __________
9. Dates of Military Service: From __________ to __________
10. Rank at time of test __________
11. Rank at time of discharge __________
12. D.V.A. Claim No: ________ 11. Claim Results: __________
13. Name of friend or relative who would know your address, should you move.
Name: ______________ Telephone No: (__) ____ - ______
Address: ______________________________
City: ____________ State: ________ ZIP Code: ________

PART II: Atomic/Nuclear Test Participation

14. Which of the following series of tests did you participate in?

_ 1945 Alamogordo	_ 1945 Hiroshima	_ 1945 Nagasaki
_ 1946 Crossroads	_ 1948 Sandstone	_ 1951 Ranger
_ 1951 Greenhouse	_ 1951 Buster/Jangle	_ 1952 Tumbler/Snapper
_ 1952 Ivy	_ 1953 Upshot/Knothole	_ 1954 Castle
_ 1955 Teapot	_ 1955 Wigwam	_ 1956 Redwing
_ 1957 Plumbbob	_ 1958 Plumbbob	_ 1958 Hardtack I, II
_ 1958 Argus I, II, III	_ 1961 Nougat	_ 1962 Dominic I, II
_ 1979 Enewitok Cleanup		

_ Other Tests: Dates__________ Name______________________
Description______________________________
15. Ship/Unit/Duties during tests______________________

Please use additional sheets of paper to give full details for each shot and exposure to ionizing radiation in activities other than testing.
16. Dates in the test area(s). (M/D/Y) From: ________ to ________
17. Were you issued: Film Badge Yes _ No _ ; Dosimeter Yes _ No _
Protective Clothing Yes __ No __; Radiac Meter Yes __ No __
18. Approximate total time of your exposure to radiation _____ (days)

-2-

Part III: Health/ Medical Information.

19. During the first six weeks after exposure, did you suffer any of the following medical problems? Please check as many as apply. Check twice if you received medical treatment for any of the conditions listed:

_ Rashes _ Nausea _ Vomiting _ Redness of Skin
_ Loss of Hair _ Diarrhea _ Nerves _ Fatigue/Apathy
_ Bleeding gums ___ Other ____________

20. If you were treated for any medical problems during the first few weeks after the test detonation(s), If you can, please name the Location/Unit/Doctor/Medical Problem, etc. Please give all the particulars you can remember: ____________

21. Do you currently have, or have you had in the past, any of the following medical problems:

_ Cataracts _ Loss of Teeth _ Lymphoma _ Diabetes _ Sterility
_ Polycythemia Vera _ Multiple Myeloma _ Cancer of Bile Ducts
_ Heart Attack(s) (No. ___) _ Cancer of Thyroid _ Breast Cancer
_ Leukemia _ Cancer of Pharynx _ Cancer of Small Intestine
_ Heart Surgery _ Cancer of Esophagus _ Cancer of Pancreas
_ Cancer of Stomach _ Cancer of Gall Bladder _ Bone Cancer
_ Primary Liver Cancer _ Chromosomal Damage _ Cancer of Testes

22. Have you had a physical examination at a D.V.A. medical facility in accordance with Public Law 97-72 ? Yes _ No _

23. Do you receive benefits under:
Public Law 100-321 ? Yes _ No _ or (From D.V.A.)
Public Law 98-542 ? Yes _ No _ or (From D.V.A.)
Public Law 101-426? Yes _ No _ (From Dept of Justice)

24. D.V.A. hospital you presently are being treated/ plan to be treated:

Name ____________
Address ____________
City ________ State ______ ZIP Code ______

PART IV: Family Information

25. _ Married _ Widowed _ Divorced _ Single
26. Wife's name: ____________
27. Number of children _____ Number of Grandchildren _____
28. Please furnish information on any child or grandchild who has health problems which may relate to your exposure to ionizing radiation. (Continued on page 4.)

- 3 -

PART V: Health Problems of Children and Grandchildren that may be due to veteran's exposure to ionizing radiation. [illegible] GD (Granddaughter). Check illnesses.
A. Syndromes S D GS GD ___ Down's S D GS GD ___ Turner's ___ Others S D GS GD

B. Diseases that may be due to damage to Veteran's Reproductive System
S D GS GD ___ Multiple Sclerosis S D GS GD ___ Cystic Fibrosis Others S D GS GD

C. Birth Defects (Congenital Deformations)
Abnormal Growths, Describe S D GS GD ____________

Others S D GS GD ____________
D. Learning Disabilities S D GS GD ___ Mental Retardation
S D GS GD ___ Slow Learner S D GS GD ___ Low IQ Others S D GS GD

E. Health Problems Same As Fathers or Grandfathers. Refer to p. 3.
_ Cataracts _ Loss of Teeth _ Lymphoma _ Diabetes _ Sterility
_ Polycythemia Vera _ Multiple Myeloma _ Cancer of Bile Ducts
_ Heart Attack(s) (No. ___) _ Cancer of Thyroid _ Breast Cancer
_ Leukemia _ Cancer of Pharynx _ Cancer of Small Intestine
_ Heart Surgery _ Cancer of Esophagus _ Cancer of Pancreas
_ Cancer of Stomach _ Cancer of Gall Bladder _ Bone Cancer
_ Primary Liver Cancer _ Chromosomal Damage _ Cancer of Testes
___ Others ____________

PART VI: Additional Information and Comments.

APPENDIX C

Epidemiology Primer

Begin with a question such as "Does exposure X cause disease Y?" The premise of epidemiology is so deceptively simple that it can be described in two sentences:

- Scientists compare two groups of people that are alike in all ways except that one group was exposed to X and the other group was not.
- If more people in the exposed group than in the other group have the disease, Y, scientists have an epidemiologic clue that exposure X may be harmful. (Note: We have not proven that X causes Y; we have shown that in this sample X and Y occur together more often than we would have expected them to by chance.)

What, however, takes scores of technical textbooks and fuels ongoing debates are the "how to" and "what if," "buts," "on the other hands," and "howevers" that make all the difference between error-laden, error-tinged, and accurate study results. In the next few pages, we describe several known pitfalls and techniques for avoiding them. That should provide a basic background to enable non-technically oriented readers to dig into this report.

Epidemiology is the study of the distribution and determinants of disease and its effects (e.g., death) in human populations. While examining data, rather than people (as in clinical research) or animals or chemicals (as in laboratory research), epidemiologic analyses seek to understand causation. Epidemiology attempts to tease out the relationships between factors—be they characteristics of people (e.g., age, race, sex), or their work (tension-filled or relaxed, indoors

---

This text is excerpted from *Mortality of Veteran Participants in the CROSSROADS Nuclear Test,* Johnson et al. (1996).

or outdoors) or home (sufficient or insufficient food, shelter, and social support) environments; characteristics of potentially harmful factors (viruses, poverty, metabolic disturbances, high cholesterol, or radiation) or beneficial factors (including new medication, surgery, medical devices, health education, income, and housing); or measures of health status (mortality rates, cholesterol levels, or disease incidence). Notice that one factor can be at once a characteristic, risk factor, and outcome. A key distinction between epidemiologic and experimental data is that epidemiologic studies usually are not designed experiments with purebred animal subjects randomized to be exposed or not exposed. Rather, one makes use of exposure situations that have occurred for various reasons to learn what one can. This is essential in situations such as the study of CROSSROADS participation where a randomized design is impossible retrospectively.

It is important to understand that while epidemiology seeks to understand causal pathways, it cannot prove causation. Epidemiology uses judgment, statistics, and skepticism to reach *descriptions* and *interpretations* of relationships and associations. It is both a practical technique and an intellectual framework for considering the possibilities of causal relationships. It is the approach we have taken in this study.

Epidemiologists compare groups. The key to making sound comparisons is in choosing groups that are alike in all ways except for the matter being studied. This selection of comparison groups is where the science, mathematics, and art of good epidemiology are blended. For example, because age and sex are associated with health risks and conditions, data regarding age and sex are collected, making it possible in the analysis to either compare like age distributions and sexes or statistically adjust the data to account for known differences.

CHOICE OF COMPARISON GROUP

In studying CROSSROADS participants, comparison group options include the development of a specific control group, internal comparisons by level of exposure, and use of national statistics. Each carries useful and restrictive elements.

If, for example, one wants to study the effect of something on lung cancer, knowing what we do about cigarette smoking and lung cancer, we would want to pick two groups to compare that do not differ in smoking practices, for that difference could mask the true causal relationship we are looking to explore. In studies of military participants, it helps to use a reference group that is also military. After checking age and sex, we rest a bit more comfortably that the two groups are rather likely to be similar on a host of unmeasured characteristics— such as smoking behavior. If, however, we chanced to compare the woodwind section of the Navy band (good breathers) with an average group of smokers, we could encounter differences attributable to smoking behavior. Closer to the concerns of this study, we would not want to compare a group exposed to nuclear test radiation with a group drawn from radiation workers. (Although if there were a few radiation workers in a much greater number of comparison group members, any possible confounding would be very diluted.)

Study results hinge on differences between the two (or more) groups compared in the study. So, choice of comparison group(s) is an extremely important task, one that has both conceptual and practical aspects. Consistent findings over hundreds of different disease-exposure inquiries demonstrate what we refer to as a "healthy worker effect." With no hypothesized harmful exposure, a cohort of workers or soldiers is *expected* to be healthier, as reflected in mortality and morbidity rates, than a general cohort. To be included in the soldier or worker cohort, the individual has to be mentally and physically functioning at or above whatever level is required for the duties of that cohort. In the extreme, those on their "deathbeds" are not hired or recruited. Furthermore, individuals are excluded from military service if they are not "fit," according to clinical and laboratory findings. Numerous studies have confirmed that this healthy worker effect is most pronounced in measurements taken close to the time of hiring (or entry into military service) but continues for decades.

Using a military comparison group addresses and avoids the healthy soldier effect but does carry other drawbacks. While government and other groups routinely gather statistics (including demographic, health, and employment descriptors) on general populations, such as U.S. males aged 45–65, data are not readily available for more finely (or even grossly) honed comparison groups in the military or elsewhere. Using a specifically designed comparison group, therefore, adds expense and time to a study. Furthermore, it increases the opportunity to introduce confounding information that could bias the findings.

Many of these difficulties can be overcome with meticulous attention to technique, innovative study designs and analytic plans, and a balanced view of what statistics do and do not say. These options are difficult to weigh for practiced scientists and no less difficult to explain to and discuss with non-technically trained readers; misunderstanding between scientist and public often occurs.

One option is to compare the group in question (for example, military personnel who participated in nuclear tests) with more than one comparison group, aiming to tease out relationships between exposure and outcome by seeing similarities and differences in those comparisons. The current CROSSROADS study is structured around a military comparison group, chosen to match on age, rank, time period, and military occupation—all available characteristics—but specifically *not* CROSSROADS test participants. Secondarily, we included statistical comparisons with the general U.S. male population.

FINE TUNING OF EXPOSED GROUP

Although "participant" vs. "nonparticipant" is an intuitively reasonable place to start analysis in this study, there are intricate details to consider. Foremost, not all "participants" received the same amount of exposure (or potential exposure, measured exposure, expected exposure, or type of exposure) as all the other participants.

We look, therefore, for some way(s) of measuring the amount of exposure and then characterizing individuals in relation to their known (or expected or hypothesized) dose (amount of exposure). Otherwise, if only a few of the participants were exposed, any effect (on cancer mortality, for example) would be diluted because most of the "exposed" were actually "not exposed" (or minimally exposed) and would not reflect the exposure-disease association. No difference would be observed and we would not know whether that meant there was indeed no difference or the comparison groups were identified in ways in which a real difference could not be observed.

Because adequate direct exposure measurements are not always available, researchers attempt to develop surrogate measures of exposure. In this study we pursued data from actual dosimetry measurements made at the time of the nuclear tests, recalculations done to address the known incompleteness of those measures, self-reports of participants, and coherent assumptions based on knowledge of radiation physics, troop logistics, on-site reportage, logs, and documents as well as logic.

CONFOUNDERS

It will come as no surprise that some characteristics—such as age and sex— are associated with numerous measures of health status. They are, also, associated with military experience in general and CROSSROADS participation in particular. These are likely confounders (things that confuse a straightforward comparison), because they are characteristics associated with both the outcome and the putative causative element under study. While a military comparison group based on broad categories of age, sex, similar unit assignment, and military rank provides some assurance of comparability, differences are still likely to exist. When we know what the confounders are *and* we can measure them, we can take them into account in the statistical analysis. Careful choice of comparison groups can help to limit the effect of unknown confounders. Chapter 10 and Chapter 11 of this report describe the design and analytic steps we took to control for potential confounding.

Examples of characteristics that frequently confound exposure-disease associations include age, race, sex, socioeconomic status, occupation, and various behaviors, such as alcohol and tobacco use. In specific studies investigators may hypothesize potential confounders such as ethnicity; military service-related exposures, including sunlight, altitude, and preventive and therapeutic attention to infectious disease, as well as the diseases themselves; and other risks based on lifestyle, geography, and postmilitary careers.

DATA COLLECTION

Once researchers have chosen the groups to study, avoiding the pitfalls—or at least, recognizing and measuring them as best as possible for later adjustment, they face a new set of problems during the planning and conduct of data collection. If you plan to get information directly from the subject, you need to do all you can to find all subjects, regardless of their being in the case/participant or control/comparison group and regardless of the outcome under study. If you are getting information from records, you need to get records for all subjects, again regardless of their being in the case/participant or control/comparison group and regardless of the outcome under study.

For example, if you are attempting to get information from subjects themselves and want to find out mortality rates and gather information by phone, *you will not find anyone to be dead.* Conversely, if you look only at death certificates, *you will not find anyone alive.* These somewhat tongue-in-cheek extremes are easy to avoid; the shades of gray around and between them, however, are often stumbling blocks in data collection and then analysis and interpretation. The reasons are that there are biases in record systems: not all records have an equal likelihood of being retrieved. For example, in looking at hospital records, specific cases involved in lawsuits may be in the general counsel's office and not in the clinic's file, where they would normally be found. There are also mundane reasons for all data not being equally available: records can be lost or destroyed, intentionally or unintentionally, by flood or fire, as in the case of veterans' records at the National Personnel Records Center in St. Louis (see Chapter 7). Note that bias does not necessarily mean prejudicial treatment, but would include any process that systematically treats one set of records differently than another.

To minimize possible biases, a number of general rules and protocols have evolved to guide researchers—regardless of participant or comparison group and regardless of likely outcome. These protocols include developing an understanding of all data sources and how they may be expected to affect data distributions and establishing clear decision rules. A summary list of rules could include:

- ensuring that there is an equal likelihood of finding records of people in each group; if a source of data is available for only one group, do not use it.
- being aware of biases built into record systems. There are potentially many of these: people with illness are more likely to seek care; veterans with lower incomes or service-connected disabilities are more likely to seek VA care; care-seeking behavior varies over time (for example, as VA benefits change); medical record technologies change; whether patients or family members have concerns about benefits or suspicions of causation could influence whether they notify the recordkeeping agency; data may be missing due to circumstances beyond human control, such as a fire destroying paper files; and data accuracy is associated with level of ascertainment, such as completeness of fact-of-death, date-of-death, or cause-of-death information.

- using a firm cut-off date for the follow-up period. It is necessary to treat participants and comparisons equally when it comes to data collection, followup, and maintenance. The decisions made should be definable. Researchers should examine—according to biologic, logistical, and cost implications— choices involving latency periods, cohort age, or pending compensation questions. Once cut-offs are chosen, it is best to recognize and honor the choice (although it may seem arbitrary in practice).
- recognizing that raw numbers offer different information than do rates or proportions. The latter include a context for interpreting the importance of the raw number. While reporting the number of people dead is often informative, it is insufficient to use *percentages* without first identifying a conceptually acceptable denominator and then using the *entire* denominator in any calculation. For example, when examining constructs such as "average age at death," one should account for the amount of time available for observations since the average will change over time as larger proportions of the sample die. For example, let's follow the mortality experience of a hypothetical sixth-grade class of 25 students in 1923. Looking at them in 1925, after one 13-year-old died in a motor vehicle accident, we would see an average age at death of 13 years. If no one else in that class were to die over the next 15 years, then, in 1940, the average age at death would still be 13 because all members of the cohort who had died (in this case one person) did so at age 13. By 1975 (the original children would now be about 61 years old), perhaps another 10 had died; the average age at death would be higher than 13, but necessarily lower than 61. The average would depend on when the deaths occurred within that period. The average age of death calculated at any point in time is the average of the ages at death for all members deceased by that point in time. The average will change over time as more deaths are added into the calculations. The average does not reflect the total mortality experience of the group until *all* members have died. Statistical techniques have been developed to even out such things, so that numbers can be compared meaningfully.

These comments show the bridges among data collection, reporting, and analysis. In the following sections, we continue with analysis issues.

INTERPRETING DATA FINDINGS

Let us say that comparison groups were chosen appropriately, unbiased data collected, and one group has more disease than the other. Epidemiology provides for the use of judgment in considering whether a numerical relationship might reflect a causal one. The criteria of causal judgment—which have been stated in many contexts—involve two broad considerations: Are the exposure and the outcome *associated*? Does that association *make sense,* based on biological as well as other physical, historical, and study design factors?

Epidemiology studies are designed to describe numerical associations between factors (risks, treatments, outcomes). In interpreting the results we look at characteristics of those associations. Evidence supporting a causal association mounts if the association is consistent (observed in a variety of studies addressing the same type of exposure in different circumstances), strong (e.g., with high relative risk ratios), and specific. Statistics serve as a tool to quantify the strength of associations relative to random background fluctuations, which are more likely to be observed the smaller the sample considered. Through mathematical theory and centuries of data analysis, statisticians have derived (and continue to derive) methods to deal with multiple comparisons, effects of misclassification, inferences from samples, and combining data from diverse (but not too diverse) studies.

Vital to the epidemiologist's examination of data are the issues of statistical measures and variability. Starting with a sample of people, we generate statistical measures (or statistics, for short) that summarize some important information collected on them (e.g., death rates). Variability enters the picture when we take a particular sample, because the statistics we generate for that particular sample will be specific to that sample; a different sample would generate different statistics because the individuals in one sample are not the same as in the other. Yet, if a sample has been selected essentially at random and something is known or assumed about the distribution of the statistics generated from that particular sample, then we can make some general statements about the variability of those statistics.

Typically, we characterize a particular statistical measure's variability by quantifying how much it would vary just by taking different samples and recalculating that same statistic. In general, it turns out that the larger the sample, the smaller the variability. It is customary to calculate two limits, called the lower and upper 95 percent confidence limits, that have the property that if we repeatedly drew samples and recalculated the statistic, these different values would lie between the upper and lower confidence limits 95 times out of 100. The interval between the upper and lower confidence limits is thus called a 95 percent confidence interval. The wider the confidence interval, the more variability there is in the statistic.

It is frequently of interest to know what the variability of a statistic is because it affects its interpretation. If the mortality rates of participants and controls are equal, for example, then the ratio of these two rates (the rate ratio) should be 1.0. However, there is inherent variability in this rate ratio statistic, so that we want to calculate its 95 percent confidence interval. If the ratio is only slightly more than or less than 1.0, for example, by an amount that lies within the confidence interval, we customarily conclude that this small deviation from 1.0 could be attributed to inherent variability (chance), such as that which comes from selecting different samples. On the other hand, if the confidence interval for the rate ratio does not include 1.0, its value is not attributed to chance and it is considered statistically significant.

Another way to determine whether a particular statistic (let us stick to rate ratios) is bigger or smaller than 1.0 is to perform a statistical test. A statistical test is a more formal statistical procedure that computes a statistic under the assumption that some null hypothesis is true. A typical null hypothesis might be: there is *no* difference in mortality rate between group A and group B (in other words, the rate ratio is equal to 1.0). If the statistic is "unusual," then the null hypothesis is rejected. The measure of "unusual" is called a *p*-value. Customarily, a p value of less than 0.05 is considered "unusual." For example, take the above null hypotheses of no difference between mortality rates in groups A and B; that is, the rate ratio is 1.0. If observed data yield an actual rate ratio of 1.5, for instance, and an associated test statistic with a p-value less than 0.05, then we reject the null hypothesis and conclude that such a high risk ratio is unlikely (only 5 times out of 100) to be due to chance.

Finally, we need to examine a little more what "unlikely to be due to chance" means in a larger context. By custom, a value is called statistically significant if the operation of chance will produce such a value only about 5 times in 100. However, just as in the case of repeated samples, repeated analyses of different data (for example, death rates due to cancer, to heart disease, to respiratory disease, etc.), every one involving a statistical test, will carry an individual 5 percent risk of labeling a statistic significant when its increased or decreased value was actually due to chance.

Moreover, if we do many such analyses, that 5 percent risk for each one mounts up. For example, if one does 20 statistical tests of rate ratios, it is quite likely that there will be at least one rate ratio labeled statistically significant just by the operation of chance. This analytic problem is known as the multiple comparisons problem.

Because the greater the number of statistical tests, the more findings are labeled statistically significant due to chance, efforts are made to limit the number of statistical tests. This is usually done by specifying in advance a relatively small number of tests, directed at a limited number of research questions. Nevertheless, there are also times—for example, when one is interested in completely describing all the data, say, looking at a complete list of causes of death, whether or not one suspects that any of these rates are elevated—when many independent tests are made. In these situations, it is especially important to keep in mind the possibility that statistically significant rate ratios may be labeled so merely due to chance.

At the same time, one must consider that a true association may fail to test as statistically significant by chance or because of lack of statistical power. The power of a study to detect a real association (if there were one) depends on sample size, the incidence of the outcome in the absence of exposure, and the strength of association between the exposure and the outcome.

In considering whether an observed association makes sense causally, epidemiologists consider the temporal relationship between the factors (e.g., if described appropriately, an outcome cannot precede a cause), the biologic plausibility of the association, and its coherence with a range of other related knowledge (radiation biology, for example). No one of these factors is necessar ily sufficient to prove causation. In fact, causation cannot actually be proven; it can only be supported (weakly or strongly) or contradicted (weakly or strongly).

Epidemiology uses numbers, going to extreme lengths at times to "split hairs" and "search under rocks," yet relies on judgment for interpretation. It is hoped that the considered judgments of epidemiologists will be useful to the judgment of clinicians in making treatment decisions and of policymakers in making legislation and regulatory and procedural decisions.

EPIDEMIOLOGY SUMMARY RELATED TO THIS STUDY

This is a report of a retrospective cohort study comparing military participants in CROSSROADS with military nonparticipants who are similar in age, rank-rating, military occupation, time frame of service, and sex. To more accurately measure exposure, we developed and used criteria for those participants most likely to have been more highly exposed. The study design calls for tight controls on the selection process for assignment to participant or comparison groups, data access, and data follow-up.

The endpoints considered are mortality rates. Specific causes of death were chosen based on understanding of disease process and *a priori* expectations based on knowledge and suspicion of radiation effects.

This study will *not* say whether Private Rogers, Rodriguez, or Rosenthal died of cancer because of Operation CROSSROADS. It *may* be able to say that the rate of cancer among all CROSSROADS participants was—or was not—different from the rate of cancer among comparable nonparticipants. Whether associations are reported with relative surety or uncertainty depends on the data themselves and on statistical techniques for sifting the wheat from the chaff. If this were easy, we would not still be studying and arguing about radiation effects.

The Medical Follow-up Agency of the Institute of Medicine, National Academy of Sciences, conducted the study, relying, as necessary, on records maintained by government and private groups. MFUA is itself "disinterested" in that it stands to neither lose nor gain from its findings in this study: it will neither receive nor be denied compensation, nor will it be held fiscally or programmatically responsible for such compensation or related care. Because this study (not unlike many other studies of human suffering and possible blame and responsibility) has an historical overlay of tremendous emotion and distrust, we must be especially careful to follow generally accepted ground rules for valid studies and to describe openly our rationale for various decisions throughout.

APPENDIX D

Verification of Completeness and Accuracy of the Participant Roster

In the early 1990s, the Defense Threat Reduction Agency (then the Defense Nuclear Agency) announced that the personnel dataset it had provided MFUA contained substantial errors of inclusion and exclusion. Because this dataset was the basis for MFUA's Five Series Study (FSS) published in 1985, the U.S. General Accounting Office (GAO), the congressional Office of Technology Assessment (OTA), concerned members of Congress and their staffs, and MFUA itself recommended redoing the mortality analyses using a corrected dataset. Using GAO estimates of required additions (28,215) and deletions (14,854), the correct dataset would have 59,547 participants; OTA estimates (15,000 additions and 4,500 deletions) would yield 56,686 participants. These classification errors were discovered by NTPR in the process of updating its participant database following its 1987 consolidation of the databases previously maintained by each branch of service.

Verification of the completeness and accuracy of the participant file is important to any study and of special concern for this one given its history. In Chapter 5, we describe the development of the participant cohort used in the analyses for this report. This appendix presents the detailed verification and validation work we did to assure ourselves and the reader of the validity of this roster.

We pursued two avenues of validation. The first was a comparison of the 1985 participant roster with the 1999 participant roster.[1] In the second, we compared the 1999 roster with participant lists compiled independently of the Nuclear Test Personnel Review (NTPR) database.

[1] For this chapter, we refer to the dataset on which the analyses reported in this publication are based as *the 1999 data* in keeping with the report publication date and parallel to references to *the 1985 data* for the earlier report. The datasets for each of these reports, however, were constructed and frozen prior to the reported analyses.

COMPARISON TO THE PARTICIPANT ROSTER USED FOR THE 1985 STUDY

By comparing the current participant dataset to the 1985 version (Robinette et al., 1985) and seeking verification of participation for sampled individuals, we were able to describe the differences between the two rosters and comment on the reasons for the changed counts. We did not change the 1999 participant data based on our findings of the comparison with the 1985 data. Rather, we used the information to describe the completeness of the dataset and to comment on the way any incompleteness might affect the 1999 study findings.

Computer File Match

MFUA staff created computer programs to select participant records that *matched* on the DNA lists provided for both the 1985 study and the current study. Because military service numbers are printed in varied formats, we truncated the alphabetical prefixes and added leading zeros where necessary.

- *Method A:* A match was sought for complete military service number (MSN)—looking at all four MSN fields on the R90 dataset—plus the first five characters of last name and the initial character of the first name.
- *Method B:* Matches were sought for the full first name and full last name; MSN was then checked by hand to detect similarities.

Comparing the 49,148 records in the 1985 data file (which includes clearly erroneous entries that correctly had been deleted from the cohort for the 1985 publication) and the 68,168 in the 1999 file, matches were found by methods A or B, above, for 38,729 individuals. These matching programs designated certain records as *discrepancies.* These records do not match exactly on all available variables (last name, first name, date of birth [DOB], Social Security number [SSN], military service number [MSN]) but do match on some loosely defined criteria (documented below).

Reviewing Discrepancies by Hand

Reviewing the first few pages of discrepancy lists produced by the computer matching program, we noted for each discrepant pair an opinion: match, probably a match, could be a match (not enough information), probably not a match, and not a match. Table D-1 presents the criteria we set for use in judging whether two *entries* matched.

TABLE D-1. Instructions to Staff—Common Errors

Be Alert for Common Errors Based on:	One File	Other File
Number readability problems	3 9	8 0
Letter readability problems	M D L	N P I
Adjacent-digit typing errors	9	0
Missed hyphens	MEDINADIAZ	MEDINA-DIAZ
Typist using familiar patterns	CK MAC -OR -MAN -L- BURGER	C MC- -ER -MEN -LL- BERGER
Formatting differences		
Leading zeros	00001234	1234
Ending zeros	12340000	00001234
Letters within a number string	AF42899	42899

For example, the examples from two files in Table D-2 would probably be true matches.

TABLE D-2. Instructions to Staff—Examples

Nature of Discrepancy	One File	Other File
Understandable discrepancy on DOB	241100	241105
Understandable discrepancy on SSN	123-45-6789	123-45-6780
Understandable discrepancy on MSN	765432	0000765432 7654320000 AF0765432 765482 764582

NOTE: DOB = date of birth; MSN = military service number; and SSN = Social Security number.

Once we determined whether the MSN, SSN, and DOB information from the 1985 list and the 1999 listed record matched sufficiently, we judged whether the *record* matched, using a set of decision rules arrayed in Table D-3. Thirty-six combinations were possible. The decisions noted in upper case occurred in the sample; the lower-case decisions are what we would have chosen had these combinations occurred.

APPENDIX D

TABLE D-3. Instructions to Staff—Availability and Consistency of Identification Data

Combination	MSN	SSN	DOB	Match Decision
1	x	x	x	NO
2	x	#	x	NO
3	x	x	#	NO
4	x	#	#	NO
5	x	=	~	yes
6	x	#	=	no
7	x	~	#	yes
8	x	=	x	yes
9	x	x	=	NO
10	#	x	x	no
11	#	#	x	no
12	#	x	#	no
13	#	#	#	no
14	#	=	=	yes
15	#	#	=	no
16	#	=	#	yes
17	#	=	x	yes
18	#	x	=	no
19	=	x	x	
20	=	#	x	yes
21	=	x	#	
22	=	#	#	YES
23	=	=	=	YES
24	=	#	=	yes
25	=	=	#	yes
26	=	=	x	yes
27	=	x	=	yes
28	~	x	x	
29	~	#	x	yes
30	~	x	#	
31	~	#	#	
32	~	=	=/~	YES
33	~	#	=	YES
34	~	=	#	yes
35	~	=	x	yes
36	~	x	=	YES

NOTE: DOB = date of birth; MSN = military service number; SSN = Social Security number; "=" indicates an exact match; "#" indicates one or both are missing; "x" indicates that they are different; and "~" indicates that they are very similar (with understandable discrepancy). Uppercase letters indicate decisions that occurred in the sample; lowercase letters indicate decisions that we likely would have chosen had these combinations occurred.

Using the methods described above, we reviewed three discrepancy lists:

- *Method C:* Listed all records where the first four letters of the last name and the first three letters of the first name matched, regardless of the remaining letters.
- *Method D:* Listed all records, using the first three letters of the last name and the first three letters of the first name, where first and last names were reversed.
- *Method E:* Listed all records where complete last names and complete first names were reversed.

All three lists, generated after methods A- and B-determined matches were culled, disregarded whether DOB, SSN, and MSN matched.

The first 10 pages of list C consist of possible matches involving 177 participants on the 1999 roster and 103 participants on the 1985 roster. (Numbers of records do not match because, for example, one 1985 list "Bil* Smit*" could have matched four 1999 list "Bil* Smit*"s.) Using this group as a sample, we identified 25 matches. Table D-4 shows the match results from each method's list.

TABLE D-4. Matching of Participant Names on the 1985 and 1999 Study Rosters by Types of Matching Methods Used

			Matches *		
	1985 List	1999 List	No.	% of 1985 List	% of 1999 List
Lists A + B (all)	49,148	68,168	38,729	78.8	56.8
List C (sample)	103	177	25	24.3	14.1
List D (sample)	44	136	1	2.3	0.7
List E (sample)	23	24	20	87.0	83.3

*Based on staff judgment.

Sample for DTRA Verification

We drew a sample of 50 participants from each of the five series for each of the following categories:

- participants who were found in both the 1985 participant list and the current, 1999, participant list, were called *matched;*
- participants who are currently in the study but could not be matched to a 1985 participant were called *new only;*
- participants who were in the study in 1985 but could not be matched to a participant in the 1999 file, were called *old only.*

MFUA requested documentation from the Defense Threat Reduction Agency (DTRA) to verify the status of each of the selected individuals.

Participants Found Only in the Current Dataset—New Only

Among the sample of 250 new-only participants whose names were on the 1999 list but not found in the 1985 data, 239 were confirmed as appropriately included new participants. For nine individuals, documentation found during the validation process indicated that the individuals should have been deleted from the 1999 dataset. These were deleted subsequent to the submission of the list to DTRA, but before the verification research had been completed. For one participant, classified as an error, the verification research provided a dosimetry record for an individual that indicated participation; however, the serial number belonged to another participant. No personnel records were found to confirm participation of either the named individual or the participant whose serial number was assigned to the name listed.

In summary, the review of the sample of 250 participants added to the 1999 roster (new only) found 248 to be in the correct status in the current dataset (99 percent), one erroneously still included, and one of indeterminate status (considered an error).

Participants Found in Both the 1985 and 1999 Datasets—Matched

Of the 250 matched participants for whom we requested DTRA documentation, 247 were verified as participants. One was a verified deletion who had not yet been posted when the validation sample was sent. Two were errors:

1. an individual who was found to have left the test site 3 weeks before the shot he was thought to have attended, and
2. another who had previously been identified as a crew member of a participating ship prior to the test series, but a detailed review of the ship's records during the test found no evidence he was actually there.

Participants Found Only in the 1985 Dataset—Old Only

Of the sample of 250 participants found on the 1985 list, but not matched to a name on the 1999 participant list, 125 (50 percent) were discovered actually to be represented on the 1999 list, but the match had been obscured by inaccurate or missing identification information on one or both lists. They were recognized as matches when identification information (spelling of name or service number) was corrected during clean-up of the dataset. Another comparably sized group of 119 (48 percent) were confirmed deletions; records demonstrated that the individuals did not meet the definition of a participant. There were six errors:

- Two of the 250 were not included in the 1999 dataset but should have been.
- One had no documentation.
- Two were aboard contaminated ships after the operation but during the official post-operational period and should not have been dropped from the participant list.
- One was thought to be a civilian and dropped from the list, although later research found him to be in the military and therefore meeting participant cohort criteria.

In summary, 244 (98 percent) of the old-only group had been appropriately handled in developing the 1999 dataset.

Overlap of the 1985 and 1999 Participant Rosters

Eighty-four percent of the individuals included in the 1985 analysis (38,729 out of 46,186) are also included in the 1999 list. However, these people comprise only 57 percent of the 1999 list. If the 3,736 personnel whose qualifying service was only during the post-operational period (see Chapter 5) were excluded from this calculation because they reflect a change in the inclusion criteria since the construction of the 1985 list, rather than identification errors, there is still a 60 percent carryover. Table D-5 displays the extent of overlap between the 1985 and 1999 datasets.

TABLE D-5. Comparison of Current (1999) Five Series Participant Dataset and 1985 Dataset

	1985	1999[a]	Comment
Match	38,729	38,729	Participants in both studies
Old only	8,877	NA	Not now considered participants
New only[b]	NA	27,897	Newly found participants
Problem IDs	1,542	1,542	Insufficient data to positively identify
Old only + matches	47,606	NA	Size of the 1985 study (except problems)
New only + matches	NA	66,626	Size of the current study (except problems)
Total	49,148	68,168	Total size including problem records

NOTE: NA = not applicable.

[a] This validation study was done by Medical Follow-up Agency staff with a preliminary participant list; the numbers do not match the participant counts reported in the report analyses.
[b] Includes 3,736 post-onlys (change in criteria accounts for mismatch, not error in the 1985 data).

COMPARISON OF 1999 PARTICIPANT ROSTER WITH OTHER SOURCES

National Association of Atomic Veterans (NAAV) Mortality Study List

Estimating the number of persons erroneously left out of the 1999 participant list was more difficult than verifying the participation of those whose names were already known to be on the list. To estimate the rate of incorrect exclusions—that is, the proportion of actual five series participants who have been incorrectly excluded from the 1999 list—we needed to find an independent list of putative participants. We used three sources to find these additional participants.

NAAV provided us with a list of veterans (n = 1,859) who reported service in at least one of the five series. Using this list as a benchmark, we estimated a false negative rate by matching the NAAV participants against those in our current dataset, according to the criteria presented above. NAAV participants were classified as either "matches" or "insufficient data."

The NAAV database was compiled by Mr. Boley Caldwell, director, NAAV Medical History Survey, from a number of medical surveys that NAAV conducted of its members. The latest questionnaire was circulated in 1992 and has been documented elsewhere (Johnson, 1996). For this validation study, we accepted the NAAV database as it was presented to us, editing only as necessary to ensure consistency of format in fields such as date of birth and to eliminate obvious duplicate records and records of confirmed civilians. We have not attempted to contact individual veterans to verify or obtain additional identifying information.

The NAAV benchmark represents a highly selected population because it is based on health surveys that were intended to determine potentially radiogenic mortality and morbidity among atomic veterans. It is conceivable that veterans in the database may have been more likely to have contacted the NTPR program or the VA and, consequently, are more likely to be on our list of participants. To avoid this possible bias, we also sought participants through sources that were not connected with NAAV.

Of the 1,784 individual veterans in the NAAV Medical Survey who indicated participation in at least one of the five series, we were able to match all but 195 (10.9 percent) to our current participant list. We provided the identifying information on these 195 individuals to DTRA, requesting verification of participant status. Searching service records, morning reports, unit diaries, and dosimetry records, DTRA traced the participation status of all but 31. Table D-6 shows the results of the MFUA and DTRA matching processes.

Participants Solicited Through Veterans' Journals—Write-Ins

In order to obtain a group of veterans for comparison who were not associated with NAAV, we placed announcements of the MFUA studies of nuclear test participants in several veterans' publications.[2] The periodicals that published our announcement (in some form) included the following:

- *Journal of the Veterans of Foreign Wars,*
- *Journal of the American Legion,*
- *Journal of the Retired Enlisted Association,*
- *Journal of Retired Officers Association,* and
- *NAAV Newsletter.*

With the exception of the *NAAV Newsletter*, we were limited to a few lines of text inviting a response from five series veterans. The publications edited the announcement to suit their needs for format and availability of space. The NAAV accommodated us with a half-page form for its readers to fill out and send in. This enabled us to distinguish between respondents who were newsletter recipients, and most likely members of NAAV, and those who were not.

We asked veterans to provide us with personal identification information and details of their nuclear test participation. We refer to this as the *write-in* verification sample. Because the readership of these journals is broader than the NAAV survey, which was targeted to veterans who were already concerned about their health, this write-in sample probably constitutes a less selected (and potentially less biased toward illness) comparison group. Because more data were available for individuals in the *write-in* group, we were able to classify them in more detail when we matched them to the 1999 participant file:

- "Matches" corresponded to individuals in the NTPR participant file as defined above.
- "Not-five series" included individuals who mentioned the Five Series Study in their correspondence but provided documentation of participation (1) that definitely placed them at a different time and place—most often in another atomic test or (2) as civilian personnel.
- "Insufficient information" describes those individuals who did not provide enough information to classify them into one of the above categories. Typically, these responders provided only last name and initials or a nickname, with no other identifying information.

---

[2] We also asked for responses from veterans who participated in the CROSSROADS series.

TABLE D-6. Summary of Completeness of the Nuclear Test Personnel Review Participant List as Indicated by Data Collected by the National Association of Atomic Veterans (NAAV) Health Survey

Match Category	MFUA	DTRA	Total	% of Records (*n* = 1,859)	% of Military Individuals (*n* = 1,784)
Total matched	1,600	34	1,634	87.9	91.6
Duplicates or civilians	64	11	75	4.0	—
Confirmed service elsewhere, not five series[a]	—	111	111	6.0	6.2
Newly identified participants	—	8	8	0.4	0.4
Insufficient information[b]	195[c]	31	31	1.7	1.7
Total records submitted by NAAV	1,859	195[c]	1,859	100.0	100.0

NOTE: DTRA = Defense Threat Reduction Agency; MFUA = Medical Follow-up Agency.

[a] These individuals were assigned duties elsewhere during the time periods of the series in which they noted participation. Several were found at tests other than those in the five series.
[b] Personnel records could not be found for these individuals to verify or disallow participation.
[c] MFUA asked DTRA to investigate 195 records.

SOURCE: National Association of Atomic Veterans Health Survey (see Appendix B).

The amount of information provided by those who responded to our inquiry varied widely. Some veterans provided detailed documentation of their participation, including both official government documents and their own narrative description of events they witnessed. Others provided only their name and a statement that they were present at one of the five series.

In all, we received 531 responses that mentioned tests of the five series in one way or another. When we matched the respondents to our participant list, we obtained the results shown in Table D-7. We submitted to NTPR the 45 records with insufficient documentation for us to identify a match on the 1999 dataset. NTPR was able to confirm as participants or nonparticipants 40 of these individuals.

Participants from Public Meetings

In June 1993, when this study was at an early period of development, we held an open meeting. Members of the public, including atomic veteran representatives, and government officials were invited to attend. Many of the atomic veterans who were unable to attend in person provided written statements describing their involvement with the aboveground nuclear test program. We compiled a list of the subset of veterans who noted participation in at least one of the five series (n = 97) and compared them to participants on the 1999 list. We refer to this as the *public meeting* verification group. DTRA was able to identify as participants or nonparticipants all five individuals whom we could not (see Table D-8).

DISCUSSION

Comparison of the 1985 and 1999 NTPR-based participant rosters confirms the 1991 reports of substantial misclassification of participant status in the older roster. Carefully researching 250-member samples of individual records for each of the three possible comparison results—old only, new only, both (matched)—we identified four people on the 1999 list who do not meet participant cohort criteria (two of whom were also on the 1985 list) and five people listed in 1985 who were erroneously not included on the 1999 list (see Table D-9, page 181).

Applying these sample rates (2 out of 250, 2 out of 250, and 5 out of 250) to the entire old only, matched, and new only records, we estimated errors of inclusion and omission in the 1999 dataset.

TABLE D-7. Completeness of the Nuclear Test Personnel Review Participant List as Indicated by Veteran Responses to Solicitations in Veterans' Publications

Match Category	MFUA	DTRA	Total	% of Records (*n* = 531)	% of Military Individuals (*n* = 510)
Total matched	474	12	486	91.5	95.3
Duplicates or civilians	12	9	21	4.0	—
Confirmed service elsewhere, not five series[a]	—	17	17	3.2	3.3
Newly identified participants	—	2	2	0.4	0.4
Insufficient information[b]	45[c]	5	5	0.9	1.0
Total write-in records submitted	531	45[c]	531	100.0	100.0

NOTE: DTRA = Defense Threat Reduction Agency; MFUA = Medical Follow-up Agency.

[a] These individuals were assigned duties elsewhere during the five series participation period noted. Several were found at tests other than the five series.
[b] Personnel records could not be found for these individuals to verify or disallow participation.
[c] MFUA asked DTRA to investigate 45 records.

SOURCE: Veteran correspondence (write-ins).

TABLE D-8. Completeness of the Nuclear Test Personnel Review Participant List as Indicated by Veteran Responses to Public Meeting Inquiries

Match Category	MFUA	DTRA	Total	% of Records (*n* = 97)	% of Military Individuals (*n* = 90)
Total matched	85	4	89	91.8	98.9
Duplicates or civilians	7	0	7	7.2	—
Confirmed service elsewhere, not five series[a]	—	1	1	1.0	1.1
Newly identified participants	—	0	0	0.0	0.0
Insufficient information[b]	5[c]	0	0	0.0	0.0
Total write-in records submitted	97	5[c]	97	100.0	100.0

NOTE: DTRA = Defense Threat Reduction Agency; MFUA = Medical Follow-up Agency.

[a] These individuals were assigned duties elsewhere during the five series participation period noted. Several were found at tests other than the five series.
[b] Personnel records could not be found for these individuals to verify or disallow participation.
[c] MFUA asked DTRA to investigate 5 records.

SOURCE: Public meeting submissions.

TABLE D-9. Estimated Errors of Inclusion and Omission in the 1999 Dataset

Group	No. in Group	Sample Error Rate	Estimated Errors
New only	27,897	2/250 (0.8%)—in 1999 dataset who should not be	223.2
Matched	38,729	2/250 (0.8%)—in 1999 dataset who should not be	309.8
Old only	8,877	5/250 (2.0%)—should be in 1999 but are not	177.5

We then added information from three participant-identifying sources external to NTPR—the NAAV mortality study, veteran correspondence solicited by MFUA in veterans' publications, and veteran correspondence invited by MFUA in conjunction with its public meeting at the beginning of the Five Series Study. Ten individuals were confirmed by NTPR as five series participants who had not been included in its 1999 participant roster. For another 36 individuals who reported being five series participants, NTPR could neither confirm nor dismiss participant status because military records could not be found and other data sources, such as unit logs and dosimetry records, did not list these individuals. If we assume one extreme—that all 36 actually were five series participants—then there are 46 missed participants identified from non-NTPR sources (see Table D-10).

Comparing the validation information from both approaches provides evidence that the roster on which the analyses reported here are based has very few errors of omission or inclusion.

- All 533 estimated wrong inclusions constitute less than 1 percent (0.8%) of the 1999 participant cohort.
- All 46 veterans whom NTPR could not confirm as nonparticipants, plus the 178 individuals from the 1985 comparisons assessed to be wrong omissions, would add less than 1 percent (0.3%) to the 1999 participant cohort.

CONCLUSION

The participant roster on which the 1999 Five Series Study is based includes more than 99 percent of the military personnel who participated in any of the five series.

TABLE D-10. Nuclear Test Personnel Review (NTPR) Compared to Other Sources

	NAAV		Write-Ins		Public Meeting		Total	
	No.	%	No.	%	No.	%	No.	%
Participants newly identified, not included on NTPR roster	8	0.4	2	0.4	0	—	10	0.4
Insufficient information	31	1.7	5	1.0	0	—	36	1.5
Total possible missed	39	2.2	7	1.4	0	—	46	1.9

NOTE: NAAV = National Association of Atomic Veterans.

APPENDIX E

Additional Analyses

The data compiled in connection with this study are numerous and varied; they hold more information than the design of this study could absorb. In this appendix, we first provide some greater detail of cohort characteristics (Table E-1, Table E-2, Table E-3 to Table E-4). We then present the results of descriptive analyses and discuss their possible use in explaining relationships between participation and mortality.

DETAIL BY COHORT

We created four categories of paygrade to ensure groups of sufficient size for valid analysis. In Table E-1, we present the individual paygrade-level distribution by cohort.

In the absence of military occupation information, the analysis attempted to explore whether the type of unit to which the participant and referent cohort individuals were assigned could be developed as an exposure proxy. Although this was not possible, the balance of unit types across the cohorts, shown in Table E-2, helps to ensure some control for hazardous exposures (other than radiation) that military personnel routinely face in their assignments.

DETAIL BY SERVICE AND BY SERIES

Later in this appendix, we present findings from exploratory analyses of series- and service-specific hazard rations. Table E-3 and Table E-4 display the distribution of cohort member age and paygrade by selection series and branch of service.

TABLE E-1. Cohort Member Characteristics: Paygrade

	Participants (n = 68,168)		Referents (n = 64,781)		Total (n = 132,949)	
Paygrade	No.	%	No.	%	No.	%
E1	199	0.3	223	0.3	422	0.3
E2	6,471	9.5	6,034	9.3	12,505	9.4
E3	18,397	27.0	18,504	28.6	36,901	27.8
E4	11,976	17.6	12,015	18.6	23,991	18.0
E5	8,165	12.0	7,785	12.0	15,950	12.0
E6	4,833	7.1	4,647	7.2	9,480	7.1
E7	3,381	5.0	3,298	5.1	6,679	5.0
E8	6	0.0	1	0.0	7	0.0
E9	3	0.0	0	—	3	0.0
W1	240	0.4	206	0.3	446	0.3
W2	268	0.4	172	0.3	440	0.3
W3	41	0.1	40	0.1	81	0.1
W4	22	0.0	11	0.0	33	0.0
O1	1,417	2.1	1,551	2.4	2,968	2.2
O2	2,490	3.7	2,469	3.8	4,959	3.7
O3	3,378	5.0	3,612	5.6	6,990	5.3
O4	2,612	3.8	2,161	3.3	4,773	3.6
O5	2,187	3.2	1,290	2.0	3,477	2.6
O6	1,276	1.9	688	1.1	1,964	1.5
O7	162	0.2	37	0.1	199	0.1
O8	148	0.2	20	0.0	168	0.1
O9	13	0.0	3	0.0	16	0.0
O10	10	0.0	2	0.0	12	0.0
Missing	473	0.7	12	0.0	485	0.4

SERIES-SPECIFIC ASSOCIATIONS

We display the data for all three endpoints separately by test series, by service branch, and by paygrade. For leukemia only, for which our study results were most interesting, we did a formal analysis of the heterogeneity of risks among test series. We fit a baseline model including a variable that represented the number of the five series in which an individual participated: 0 (for refer ents), and 1 to 5 for participants. We then fit a model with five dummy variables, one variable for participation (yes or no) in each of the series. The difference in fit (assessed by log likelihoods) between these two nested models represents a formal test of the heterogeneity in leukemia risk between series. After adjusting for the number of non-five series tests, the difference in fit between these two models was 7.19, distributed as a χ^2 with 4 degrees of freedom. The associated probability is .13, indicating a lack of significant difference in leukemia risk among the five test series.

Notwithstanding this lack of a statistically significant difference in leukemia risk among the five series, we decided to undertake further investigations to identify subgroups with high leukemia risk. Part of the reason for this decision was to investigate further the significant excess risk among land series participants (see below). However, we must acknowledge that the identification of high-risk subgroups is a pursuit fraught with difficulty; because there is no clear statistical evidence of differences, one may well be studying only statistical noise (i.e., expected random variation). However, it should also be noted that formal statistical tests of heterogeneity tend to have little statistical power.

Table E-5 shows standardized mortality ratios (SMRs) and hazard ratios for the three primary mortality endpoints (all cause, all malignancies, and leukemia*) by test series. SMR ratios are significantly less than 1.0 for all-cause mortality in series UPSHOT-KNOTHOLE and PLUMBBOB. The corresponding relative hazard for UPSHOT-KNOTHOLE is significantly less than 1.0, whereas the one for PLUMBBOB is not. In test series REDWING, all-cause and all-malignancy hazard ratios are significantly greater than 1.0.

Although none of the SMR ratios or relative hazards for leukemia is significantly different from 1.0, the values are highest for series UPSHOT-KNOTHOLE, CASTLE, and PLUMBBOB. The SMR ratio for leukemia for the GREENHOUSE series is low, partly because the SMR for participants is low, but mostly because the SMR for referents is high, relative to all of the other series.

Table E-6 shows similar data by service branch. Other than all-cause mortality among Air Force and Army servicemen (which is significantly lower among participants), no other SMR ratios are significantly different from 1.0. Marines show the highest SMR ratios for all three mortality endpoints, compared to other service branches, and it appears that these ratios are elevated because participant SMRs are high, rather than referent SMRs being low.

*ICD-9 codes 204 through 208 apply to types of leukemia. In these analyses, based on current understanding of leukemia radiogencity, we exclude chronic lymphoid leukemia (ICD-9 code 204.1) from the grouping identified as leukemia.

TABLE E-2. Cohort Member Characteristics: Type of Military Unit

	Participants (n = 68,168)		Referents (n = 64,781)		Total (n = 132,949)	
Unit Category	No.	%	No.	%	No.	%
ADMIN	4,948	7.3	4,202	6.5	9,150	6.9
AIRDEF	78	0.1	180	0.3	258	0.2
AIRDEVCEN	49	0.1	256	0.4	305	0.2
AIRDIV	47	0.1	45	0.1	92	0.1
ANTITANK	0	—	3	0.0	3	0.0
ARMOR	943	1.4	766	1.2	1,709	1.3
ARTILLERY	3,646	5.4	3,513	5.4	7,159	5.4
AVIATION	2,592	3.8	3,082	4.8	5,674	4.3
BASE	4,817	47.1	2,307	3.6	7,124	5.4
BATTALION	125	0.2	111	0.2	236	0.2
BOMB	559	0.8	767	1.2	1,326	1.0
CAMP/STA	15	0.0	2	0.0	17	0.0
CARGO	853	1.3	795	1.2	1,648	1.2
CARRIER	1,814	2.7	2,948	4.6	4,762	3.6
CENTER	141	0.2	112	0.2	253	0.2
COMBAT	2,568	3.8	2,439	3.8	5,007	3.8
COMMAND	1,199	1.8	1,362	2.1	2,561	1.9
COMPANY	287	0.4	259	0.4	546	0.4
COMSTAF	2,317	3.4	1,929	3.0	4,246	3.2
CONTROL	323	0.5	825	1.3	1,148	0.9
DESTROYR	2,432	3.6	2,397	3.7	4,829	3.6
DETACHMT	8	0.0	7	0.0	15	0.0
ENGINEER	1,340	2.0	1,374	2.1	2,714	2.0
ESCORT	664	1.0	537	0.8	1,201	0.9
FIGHTER	370	0.5	307	0.5	677	0.5
FORT	26	0.0	0	—	26	0.0
HELO	486	0.7	245	0.4	731	0.6
HQTRS	890	1.3	837	1.3	1,727	1.3
INFANTRY	5,322	7.8	5,582	8.6	10,904	8.2
LAB	94	0.1	76	0.1	170	0.1

LCRAFT	1,237	1.8	1,209	1.9	2,446	1.8
MAINT	51	0.1	199	0.3	250	0.2
MAPCHART	0	—	21	0.0	21	0.0
MATERIEL	319	0.5	315	0.5	634	0.5
MEDICAL	939	1.4	1,240	1.9	2,179	1.6
MISC	181	0.3	8	0.0	189	0.1
OPERATION	241	0.4	85	0.1	326	0.3
ORDNANCE	75	0.1	66	0.1	141	0.1
REPAIR	55	0.1	142	0.2	197	0.2
SALVAGE	445	0.7	258	0.4	703	0.5
SERVICE	4,634	6.8	3,882	6.0	8,516	6.4
SIGNAL	2,968	4.4	2,794	4.3	5,762	4.3
SQUADRON	3	0.0	167	0.3	170	0.1
STORESHIP	808	1.2	843	1.3	1,651	1.2
SUBMARINE	236	0.4	91	0.1	327	0.3
TACTICAL	226	0.3	449	0.7	675	0.5
TANKERS	3,229	4.7	2,956	4.6	6,185	4.7
TECHNICAL	3,155	4.6	2,155	3.3	5,310	4.0
TENDERS	4,358	6.4	4,421	6.8	8,779	6.6
TEST	636	0.9	198	0.3	834	0.6
TRAINING	246	0.4	389	0.6	635	0.5
TRANSPORT	2,866	4.2	3,435	5.3	6,301	4.7
TUGS	879	1.3	555	0.9	1,434	1.1
UNKNOWN	765	1.1	893	1.4	1,658	1.3
WEATHER	663	1.0	654	1.0	1,317	1.0
WING	0	—	91	0.1	91	0.1

TABLE E-3. Age at Selection Series

Age (years)	GREENHOUSE		UPSHOT-KNOTHOLE		CASTLE		REDWING		PLUMBBOB	
	P	R	P	R	P	R	P	R	P	R
Air Force										
<21	279	329	69	88	219	214	514	435	165	149
≥21 and <31	1,619	1,628	948	908	1,644	1,594	1,655	1,777	948	815
≥31 and <41	833	752	1,111	699	668	666	727	661	716	646
≥41 and <51	111	56	200	59	92	91	109	102	173	171
≥51 and <61	4	6	25	9	8	23	11	6	12	19
≥61	1	0	0	1	0	0	0	0	1	0
Missing age	0	0	0	0	0	0	3	0	0	0
Total Air Force	2,847	2,771	2,353	1,764	2,631	2,588	3,019	2,981	2,015	1,800
Army										
<21	494	304	868	813	96	116	339	295	785	786
≥21 and <31	1,230	1,303	8,833	8,323	1,248	1,178	1,289	1,349	3,029	2,953
≥31 and <41	370	427	2,372	2,777	135	155	364	350	1,842	1,327
≥41 and <51	106	122	870	1,144	38	53	138	106	1,199	609
≥51 and <61	16	37	195	293	8	8	15	24	186	124
≥61	2	0	7	8	0	2	2	2	6	4
Missing age	0	0	0	0	0	0	0	0	0	0
Total Army	2,218	2,193	13,145	13,358	1,525	1,512	2,147	2,126	7,047	5,803

Marines										
<21	12	38	265	276	98	90	85	83	847	866
≥21 and <31	53	28	1,652	1,659	160	162	107	105	935	888
≥31 and <41	6	3	304	223	36	34	48	43	292	270
≥41 and <51	5	0	32	15	1	3	4	6	40	62
≥51 and <61	0	0	9	2	2	1	1	1	6	7
≥61	0	0	0	0	0	0	0	0	0	0
Missing age	0	0	0	0	0	0	0	0	0	0
Total Marines	76	69	2,262	2,175	297	290	245	238	2,120	2,093
Navy										
<21	766	733	15	25	1,840	1,660	2,569	2,244	44	73
≥21 and <31	2,785	2,667	290	288	7,968	7,651	3,641	3,767	182	139
≥31 and <41	695	605	258	124	1,209	1,268	1,115	1,045	116	73
≥41 and <51	125	95	116	40	195	237	170	210	33	27
≥51 and <61	16	13	33	2	20	14	16	11	2	2
≥61	0	0	1	0	0	1	1	5	0	1
Missing age	0	0	0	0	0	0	0	0	0	0
Total Navy	4,387	4,113	713	479	11,232	10,831	7,512	7,282	377	315
Total all services	9,528	9,146	18,473	17,776	15,685	15,221	12,923	12,627	11,559	10,011

NOTE: P = participants; R = referents.

TABLE E-4. Paygrade Groups at Selection Series

Paygrade	GREENHOUSE		UPSHOT-KNOTHOLE		CASTLE		REDWING		PLUMBBOB	
	P	R	P	R	P	R	P	R	P	R
Air Force										
E1–E3, junior enlisted	186	186	195	195	787	784	911	911	283	283
E4–E5, midlevel enlisted	1,549	1,544	432	431	878	873	1,054	1,051	440	438
E6–E9, senior enlisted	503	501	289	288	353	348	394	392	216	216
W1–W4, warrant officer	15	15	30	20	12	11	11	11	10	9
O1–O3, company officer	391	386	644	635	370	356	449	440	540	536
O4–O6, field officer	137	181	708	190	195	207	187	176	326	313
O7–O10, general officer	0	10	45	0	29	8	8	0	8	3
Missing paygrade	2	12	10	5	7	1	5	0	192	2
Total Air Force	2,783	2,835	2,353	1,764	2,631	2,588	3,019	2,981	2,015	1,800
Army										
E1–E3, junior enlisted	796	792	4,404	4,339	770	769	1,511	1,509	2,874	2,862
E4–E5, midlevel enlisted	904	899	4,165	4,112	512	512	147	145	410	409
E6–E9, senior enlisted	221	219	1,608	1,561	104	104	228	228	624	618
W1–W4, warrant officer	20	20	109	101	16	16	9	9	152	147
O1–O3, company officer	132	130	1,275	1,642	74	73	130	127	1,094	1,211
O4–O6, field officer	128	128	1,491	1,569	43	37	108	105	1,643	553
O7–O10, general officer	13	5	74	34	4	1	11	3	76	1
Missing paygrade	4	0	19	0	2	0	3	0	174	2
Total Army	2,218	2,193	13,145	13,358	1,525	1,512	2,147	2,126	7,047	5,803

Marines										
E1–E3, junior enlisted	49	49	1,424	1,419	202	200	125	125	1,236	1,234
E4–E5, midlevel enlisted	14	14	368	362	38	38	24	24	313	312
E6–E9, senior enlisted	3	3	101	95	28	25	40	36	125	124
W1–W4, warrant officer	0	0	4	3	1	1	0	0	4	4
O1–O3, company officer	4	2	204	192	15	15	38	37	289	287
O4–O6, field officer	5	1	155	104	12	11	17	15	147	127
O7–O10, general officer	1	0	1	0	0	0	0	1	3	5
Missing paygrade	0	0	5	0	1	0	1	0	3	0
Total Marines	76	69	2,262	2,175	297	290	245	238	2,120	2,093
Navy										
E1–E3, junior enlisted	1,751	1,693	46	37	4,367	4,272	3,113	3,065	37	37
E4–E5, midlevel enlisted	1,452	1,392	109	103	4,534	4,418	2,660	2,587	138	136
E6–E9, senior enlisted	711	673	95	90	1,509	1,425	1,019	951	52	49
W1–W4, warrant officer	32	0	10	0	68	0	65	59	3	3
O1–O3, company officer	308	293	189	176	613	592	461	448	65	54
O4–O6, field officer	121	62	225	73	129	124	180	171	74	36
O7–O10, general officer	7	0	26	0	8	0	7	1	2	0
Missing paygrade	5	0	13	0	4	0	7	0	6	0
Total Navy	4,387	4,113	713	479	11,232	10,831	7,512	7,282	377	315
Total all services	9,464	9,210	18,473	17,776	15,685	15,221	12,923	12,627	11,559	10,011

NOTE: P = participants; R = referents.

TABLE E-5. Standardized Mortality Ratios (SMRs) and Hazard Ratios, by Series and Participant Status, for Selected Causes of Death

	No. of Deaths		SMR		Hazard Ratio and 95% CI—Participants Relative to Referents
Cause of Death by Series	Participants	Referents	Participants	Referents	
All Causes					
GREENHOUSE	3,274	3,152	0.78	0.80	1.00 (0.95–1.05)
UPSHOT-KNOTHOLE	5,613	5,739	0.66	0.72	0.95 (0.91–0.99)
CASTLE	3,706	3,622	0.76	0.74	1.04 (1.00–1.09)
REDWING	2,879	2,682	0.77	0.73	1.07 (1.01–1.13)
PLUMBBOB	3,026	2,462	0.64	0.69	0.97 (0.92–1.03)
All Malignancies					
GREENHOUSE	858	843	0.77	0.80	0.98 (0.89–1.08)
UPSHOT-KNOTHOLE	1,532	1,493	0.70	0.73	0.97 (0.91–1.05)
CASTLE	1,013	1,002	0.77	0.76	1.03 (0.94–1.12)
REDWING	827	725	0.84	0.74	1.14 (1.03–1.26)
PLUMBBOB	851	639	0.69	0.69	1.06 (0.95–1.18)
Leukemia Minus Chronic Lymphoid Leukemia					
GREENHOUSE	21	33	0.63	1.04	0.62 (0.36–1.06)
UPSHOT-KNOTHOLE	54	33	0.82	0.54	1.49 (0.96–2.30)
CASTLE	30	21	0.73	0.51	1.40 (0.80–2.45)
REDWING	22	24	0.70	0.77	0.91 (0.51–1.63)
PLUMBBOB	29	15	0.78	0.53	1.47 (0.78–2.76)

NOTE: CI = confidence interval.

TABLE E-6. Standardized Mortality Ratios (SMRs) and Hazard Ratios, by Branch and Participant Status, for Selected Causes of Death

	No. of Deaths		SMR		Hazard Ratio and 95% CI—Participants Relative to Referents
Cause of Death by Branch of Service	Participants	Referents	Participants	Referents	
All Causes					
Air Force	3,693	3,436	0.65	0.72	0.96 (0.92–1.01)
Army	7,818	7,870	0.70	0.75	0.96 (0.93–0.99)
Marines	1,135	998	0.79	0.74	1.08 (1.00–1.18)
Navy	5,852	5,353	0.75	0.73	1.06 (1.02–1.10)
All Malignancies					
Air Force	1,005	930	0.67	0.72	0.96 (0.88–1.05)
Army	2,103	2,032	0.73	0.75	1.00 (0.94–1.06)
Marines	334	259	0.87	0.72	1.21 (1.03–1.43)
Navy	1,639	1,481	0.79	0.75	1.06 (0.99–1.14)
Leukemias Minus Chronic Lymphoid Leukemia					
Air Force	37	24	0.83	0.62	1.26 (0.75–2.12)
Army	56	53	0.64	0.64	0.99 (0.68–1.44)
Marines	13	8	1.07	0.69	1.54 (0.64–3.72)
Navy	50	41	0.77	0.67	1.17 (0.77–1.77)

NOTE: CI = confidence interval.

Table E-7 shows data by paygrade. Except for a significantly low SMR ratio for all-cause mortality among officers, none of the SMR ratios differs from 1.0. We also see that officers, whether participants or referents, have lower SMRs than enlisted men, a finding to be expected, given the known effects of rank on mortality (Seltzer and Jablon, 1977). Subjects with unknown paygrade appear anomalous in that the SMRs of participants resemble those of officers, whereas the SMRs of referents resemble those of enlisted men. Regardless, the number of subjects with unknown paygrade is small (469 participants and 12 referents).

Investigating Leukemia Risk Among Single Series Participants

We thus began our investigation of subgroup risks by looking further at differences among the test series. Our first analysis of differences among series (Table E-5) was hampered by the fact that although the first of the five series at which a participant was present defines his "official" test series, in actuality participants could have been present at more than one of the five or indeed at other tests that were not part of the five series.

Table E-8 shows participation status by assigned series. Participants are divided into two mutually exclusive participation categories: participation at assigned series or post-series only and all other (i.e., multiple series) participation. The two land series, UPSHOT-KNOTHOLE and PLUMBBOB, are characterized by their relatively high percentage of participants who were only at their assigned series or post-series (i.e., relatively little multiple series participation). On the other hand, GREENHOUSE and REDWING have the highest multiple participation rates, with roughly one-quarter of their participants having been present at other than their assigned series or post-series.

In an attempt to get sharper estimates of leukemia and cancer mortality risk across series, we took the additional step of confining the analysis to individuals who participated only in their assigned series and at no other series. Limiting the analysis to participants who were at only one of the five series has the advantage of permitting an unconfounded comparison of mortality risks across test series, although the number of participants is reduced by roughly 15 percent, from 68,208 to 57,532. Table E-9 shows that among single series participants, the risk of leukemia mortality is elevated 25 percent or more among participants of all but two test series, GREENHOUSE and REDWING. Compared to all participants, single series participants in UPSHOT-KNOTHOLE and CASTLE had lower leukemia risks, while there was little difference for PLUMBBOB (which had the highest proportion of single series participants).

TABLE E-7. Standardized Mortality Ratios (SMRs) and Hazard Ratios, by Paygrade and Participant Status, for Selected Causes of Death

Cause of Death by Paygrade	No. of Deaths		SMR		Hazard Ratio and 95% CI—Participants Relative to Referents
	Participants	Referents	Participants	Referents	
All Causes					
Junior enlisted	4,779	4,661	0.83	0.81	1.03 (0.98–1.07)
Middle enlisted	4,972	5,065	0.83	0.84	0.99 (0.95–1.03)
Senior enlisted	3,707	3,698	0.89	0.85	1.04 (0.99–1.09)
Officer	4,923	4,229	0.49	0.53	0.94 (0.90–0.98)
Unknown	117	4	0.48	0.84	1.09 (0.36–3.28)
All Malignancies					
Junior enlisted	1,261	1,171	0.82	0.76	1.08 (0.99–1.17)
Middle enlisted	1,323	1,405	0.81	0.85	0.95 (0.88–1.02)
Senior enlisted	1,054	991	0.96	0.88	1.09 (1.00–1.19)
Officer	1,419	1,133	0.57	0.57	1.00 (0.92–1.08)
Unknown	24	2	0.39	1.54	0.26 (0.05–1.38)
Leukemias Minus Chronic Lymphoid Leukemia					
Junior enlisted	40	25	0.78	0.49	1.62 (0.98–2.67)
Middle enlisted	34	42	0.67	0.83	0.80 (0.51–1.26)
Senior enlisted	24	28	0.75	0.85	0.86 (0.50–1.48)
Officer	57	31	0.78	0.53	1.44 (0.92–2.24)
Unknown	1	0	0.54	—	—

NOTE: CI = confidence interval.

TABLE E-8. Number of Participants and Percentage by Assigned Series and Type of Participation

	Type of Participation					
	At Series or Post-Series Only		Remainder *		Total	
Assigned Series	No.	%	No.	%	No.	%
GREENHOUSE	7,134	74.9	2,394	25.1	9,528	100
UPSHOT-KNOTHOLE	16,632	90.0	1,841	10.0	18,473	100
CASTLE	12,989	82.8	2,696	17.2	15,685	100
REDWING	10,093	78.1	2,830	21.9	12,923	100
PLUMBBOB	10,684	92.4	875	7.6	11,559	100
Total	57,532	84.4	10,636	15.6	68,168	100

*That is, participation in more than one series.

TABLE E-9. Relative Hazardsa (and 95% confidence interval [CI]) for Leukemia Mortality, by Series: All Participants Versus Single Series Participantsb

	All Participants		Single Series Participants	
Series	No. of Deaths[c]	Hazard Ratio (95% CI)	No. of Deaths[c]	Hazard Ratio (95% CI)
GREENHOUSE	54	0.62 (0.36–1.06)	48	0.61 (0.33–1.12)
UPSHOT-KNOTHOLE	87	1.49 (0.96–2.30)	74	1.29 (0.82–2.05)
CASTLE	51	1.40 (0.80–2.45)	43	1.26 (0.69–2.30)
PLUMBBOB	44	1.47 (0.78–2.77)	42	1.48 (0.78–2.82)
REDWING	46	0.91 (0.51–1.63)	43	1.04 (0.57–1.91)
Land series[d]	135	1.49 (1.04–2.13)	116	1.36 (0.93–1.98)
Sea series[d]	157	0.92 (0.67–1.27)	134	0.93 (0.66–1.31)
Total	282	1.14 (0.90–1.44)	250	1.10 (0.86–1.42)

[a] Adjusted for service branch, paygrade, age at participation, age squared, and age cubed.
[b] That is, no multiple series participants.
[c] Includes referent and participant leukemia deaths; change in columns reflects change in participant death count.
[d] UPSHOT-KNOTHOLE and PLUMBBOB were land series; GREENHOUSE, CASTLE, and RED-WING were sea series.

APPENDIX F

Biographical Summaries

AUTHORS

SUSAN THAUL, Ph.D. *(Study Director),* assumed the role of study director for the last phase of the Five Series Study. With the Medical Follow-up Agency, she produced the 1999 report *Potential Radiation Exposure in Military Operations: Protecting the Soldier Before, During, and After,* and coauthored the 1996 report *Mortality of Veteran Participants in the CROSSROADS Nuclear Test.* Dr. Thaul had previously led Institute of Medicine projects in women's health, national statistics, and health services research, among others. She received a Ph.D. in epidemiology from Columbia University and an M.S. in health policy and management from Harvard University. Heading the health staff of the U.S. Senate Committee on Veterans' Affairs (then chaired by Senator Alan Cranston), Dr. Thaul developed legislation in preventive health care and research, women's health care, sexual assault services and prevention, nurse and physician pay, and health effects of environmental hazards during service. Earlier positions were with the Agency for Health Care Policy and Research; the Harlem Hospital Prevention of Prematurity Project; and the New York City Health and Hospitals Corporation, where she held successive positions leading to associate director of the New York City Emergency Medical Service.

WILLIAM F. PAGE, Ph.D., has been a senior program officer at the Medical Follow-up Agency, National Academy of Sciences, since 1986. He directs a number of studies of the health of U.S. veterans, including a study of Navy veterans exposed to microwave radiation, and is a coinvestigator on two studies of American atomic veterans. He is a fellow of the American College of Epidemiology. He received his doctorate in mathematics from the University of Miami and received postgraduate training in biostatistics at the University of North Carolina School of Public Health.

HARRIET CRAWFORD, B.S., is presently the data operations manager for the agency. She has a B.S. in computer and information science from the University of Maryland. Since she began working for the Medical Follow-up Agency in 1984, she has designed and implemented many of the agency's data collection and reporting systems. She also coauthored the Institute of Medicine report, *Mortality of Veteran Participants in the Crossroads Nuclear Test.*

HEATHER O'MAONAIGH, M.A., began working as a research assistant for the Medical Follow-up Agency in June 1998. She received a B.S. in sociology from Western Washington University and an M.A. in demography from Georgetown University.

ADVISORY COMMITTEE MEMBERS

HARVEY CHECKOWAY, Ph.D. *(Chair),* is professor with joint appointments in the Departments of Environmental Health and Epidemiology at the University of Washington School of Public Health and Community Medicine, Seattle, Washington. Dr. Checkoway received his doctorate in epidemiology from the University of North Carolina at Chapel Hill in 1978 and was research assistant professor (1979–1986) and research associate professor (1987) in the University of North Carolina Department of Epidemiology. At the University of Washington he has held faculty positions of associate professor (1987–1991) and full professor (1991–present). Since 1990, Dr. Checkoway has been director of the training grant "Environmental and Molecular Epidemiology," which is funded by the National Institute for Environmental Health Sciences. His research has focused mainly on occupational and environmental determinants of chronic diseases. Research projects for which Dr. Checkoway has been principal investigator include epidemiologic studies of cancer mortality in nuclear workers, cancer mortality in phosphate industry workers, silicosis and lung cancer in silica-exposed diatomaceous earth industry workers, lung cancer among chromate-exposed aerospace workers, reproductive hazards among lead smelter workers, and environmental and genetic risk factors for Parkinson's disease.

R. J. MICHAEL FRY, M.D., is retired from Oak Ridge National Laboratory, having been head of the Cancer Section of the Biology Division. He continues to serve as consultant to the Life Sciences Division of the laboratory and as adjunct professor at the University of Tennessee. He holds M.B., B.Ch., and M.D. degrees from the University of Dublin, Ireland. Previous appointments include senior scientist in the Division of Biology and Medicine, Argonne National Laboratory, and professor in the Department of Radiology, University of Chicago. He was editor *of Radiation Research* and continues as a consulting editor. His research focused on the effects—in particular, carcinogenesis—of ionizing and ultraviolet radiation. He is a member of the International Commission on Radiological Protection's Committee 1; National Council on Radiation Protec tion and Measurements' Committees 1, 4, 7, 75, and 88; and chairman of the National Research Council's Board on Radiation Effects Research. His awards include the Failla and Hartman medals and the Lauriston Taylor lectureship.

SAMUEL HELLMAN, M.D., is the A.N. Pritzker Distinguished Service Professor, Department of Radiation and Cellular Oncology, University of Chicago, Center for Advanced Medicine, Chicago, Illinois. Dr. Hellman previously served as Dean and A.N. Pritzker Professor of the Division of Biological Sciences and the Pritzker School of Medicine and vice president for the Medical Center; physician-in-chief of the Memorial Sloan Kettering Hospital for Cancer and Allied Diseases; the Benno C. Schmidt Chair in Clinical Oncology at Memorial Sloan-Kettering Cancer Center; and professor of radiation oncology at Cornell University Medical College. At Harvard Medical School, Dr. Hellman served as chairman of the Department of Radiation Therapy; the Alvin T. and Viola D. Fuller American Cancer Society Professor; and director of the Joint Center for Radiation Therapy. Dr. Hellman has been active in both clinical and laboratory investigation including studies of breast cancer, prostate cancer, lymphoma, and the cell kinetics of the hematopoietic system. He is the author or coauthor of some 258 scientific articles; coeditor of the standard textbook on cancer, *Cancer: Principles and Practice of Oncology,* and coeditor of "The Cancer Journal" from *Scientific American.* Dr. Hellman served as chairman of the board of Allegheny College (1987–1993), where he received his B.S. degree magna cum laude in 1955; is a fellow of the Institute of Medicine of the National Academy of Sciences and the American Association for the Advancement of Science; and is a member of the board of directors of Varian Associates, Inc., and of the board of trustees of The Brookings Institution. He has served as president of both the American Society for Therapeutic Radiology and Oncology and the American Society of Clinical Oncology. He received the 1980 Richard and Hinda Rosenthal Foundation Award for Clinical Research of the American Association of Cancer Research; the Gold Medals of both the American Society of Therapeutic Radiology and Oncology and the del Regato Foundation; the American Society of Therapeutic Radiology and Oncology Centennial Hartman Orator Medal; and the Claudius Regaud Medal of the European Society for Therapeautic Radiology and Oncology.

ELAINE RON, Ph.D., is chief of the Radiation Epidemiology Branch in the Division of Cancer Epidemiology and Genetics at the National Cancer Institute. Her research focuses on the carcinogenic effects of radiation exposure and the epidemiology of thyroid cancer. She is a consultant to the United Nations Scientific Committee on the Effects of Atomic Radiation (UNSCEAR) and an adviser to the National Council on Radiation Protection and Measurements' Committee 1–8 on Induction of Thyroid Cancer by Ionizing Radiation. She is a fellow of the American Epidemiology Society and a member of the Society for Epidemiologic Research and the Radiation Research Society. Dr. Ron holds a master's degree in health service administration from Yale University and a

Ph.D. in epidemiology from Tel Aviv University. She currently is an associate editor *of Radiation Research.*

WILLIAM G. SEIBERT, M.A., is the senior archivist at the National Archives and Records Administration's Military Personnel Records facility in St. Louis. He has worked with NARA's collections of twentieth century military personnel and medical records for 20 years and has wide knowledge of alternate record sources available for use in reconstructing military service and medical data on individuals whose records were lost in the 1973 St. Louis fire. Mr. Seibert is a member of the Academy of Certified Archivists. He holds a B.A. in history from the College of William and Mary and a B.A. and M.A. in law from the University of Oxford.

JOHN E. TILL, Ph.D. Following graduation with distinction from the U.S. Naval Academy in 1967, Dr. Till served in the U.S. Navy Nuclear Submarine Program. He has received the E.O. Lawrence Award from the U.S. Department of Energy in the field of environmental science and technology for his work in public involvement and research in dose reconstruction and the Elda E. Anderson Award from the Health Physics Society. He received his Ph.D. degree from the Georgia Institute of Technology in 1976, worked as a staff scientist at the Oak Ridge National Laboratory, and in 1977 formed Radiological Assessments Corporation. Renamed the Risk Assessment Corporation in 1998, it conducts independent research concerning environmental risk analysis for radionuclides and chemicals, playing a key role in the evolution of methodologies for environmental risk analysis. Dr. Till's scientific achievements include more than 150 publications, including editing the first textbook on radiation dose analysis, *Radiological Assessment,* and other documents that stress new approaches to apply and simplify risk analysis. Dr. Till's current work focuses on the assessment of risk from past releases of radionuclides and chemicals. He has been responsible for the dosimetry estimates in a major University of Utah epidemiologic dose reconstruction project, supported by the National Cancer Institute, and was chairman of the Technical Steering Panel that directed the Hanford Environmental Dose Reconstruction Project. In this capacity, he led an effort to actively involve the public in scientific research to determine the effects of early Hanford environmental contaminants. He is a member of Committee 4 of the International Commission on Radiological Protection and the National Council on Radiation Protection and Measurements. He also serves on numerous national and international committees and advisory groups.

CLARICE R. WEINBERG, Ph.D., is currently chief of the Biostatistics Branch at the National Institute of Environmental Health Sciences, National Institutes of Health. She is also adjunct professor in the Department of Epidemiology and the Department of Biostatistics at the University of North Carolina, Chapel Hill. She holds a master's in mathematics from Brandeis University and a Ph.D. in biostatistics from the University of Washington. Her areas of exper tise are reproductive epidemiology, modeling of human fertility, and statistical methods in epidemiology. She is a fellow of the American Statistical Association, an editor at the *American Journal of Epidemiology,* and serves on the editorial boards of *Epidemiology* and *Environmental Health Perspectives.*

F

Biographical Summaries

AUTHORS

SUSAN THAUL, Ph.D. *(Study Director),* assumed the role of study director for the last phase of the Five Series Study. With the Medical Follow-up Agency, she produced the 1999 report *Potential Radiation Exposure in Military Operations: Protecting the Soldier Before, During, and After* and coauthored the 1996 report *Mortality of Veteran Participants in the CROSSROADS Nuclear Test.* Dr. Thaul had previously led Institute of Medicine projects in women's health, national statistics, and health services research, among others. She received a Ph.D. in epidemiology from Columbia University and an M.S. in health policy and management from Harvard University. Heading the health staff of the U.S. Senate Committee on Veterans' Affairs (then chaired by Senator Alan Cranston), Dr. Thaul developed legislation in preventive health care and research, women's health care, sexual assault services and prevention, nurse and physician pay, and health effects of environmental hazards during service. Earlier positions were with the Agency for Health Care Policy and Research; the Harlem Hospital Prevention of Prematurity Project; and the New York City Health and Hospitals Corporation, where she held successive positions leading to associate director of the New York City Emergency Medical Service.

WILLIAM F. PAGE, Ph.D., has been a senior program officer at the Medical Follow-up Agency, National Academy of Sciences, since 1986. He directs a number of studies of the health of U.S. veterans, including a study of Navy veterans exposed to microwave radiation, and is a coinvestigator in two studies of American atomic veterans. He is a fellow of the American College of Epidemiology. He received his doctorate in mathematics from the University of Miami and received postgraduate training in biostatistics at the University of North Carolina School of Public Health.

HARRIET CRAWFORD, B.S., is presently the data operations manager for the agency. She has a B.S. in computer and information science from the University of Maryland. Since she began working for the Medical Follow-up Agency in 1984, she has designed and implemented many of the agency's data collection and reporting systems. She also coauthored the Institute of Medicine report *Mortality of Veteran Participants in the Crossroads Nuclear Test.*

HEATHER O'MAONAIGH, M.A., began working as a research assistant for the Medical Follow-up Agency in June 1998. She received a B.S. in sociology from Western Washington University and an M.A. in demography from Georgetown University.

ADVISORY COMMITTEE MEMBERS

HARVEY CHECKOWAY, Ph.D. *(Chair),* is professor with joint appointments in the Departments of Environmental Health and Epidemiology at the University of Washington School of Public Health and Community Medicine, Seattle, Washington. Dr. Checkoway received his doctorate in epidemiology from the University of North Carolina at Chapel Hill in 1978 and was research assistant professor (1979–1986) and research associate professor (1987) in the University of North Carolina Department of Epidemiology. At the University of Washington he has held faculty positions of associate professor (1987–1991) and full professor (1991–present). Since 1990, Dr. Checkoway has been director of the training grant "Environmental and Molecular Epidemiology," which is funded by the National Institute for Environmental Health Sciences. His research has focused mainly on occupational and environmental determinants of chronic diseases. Research projects for which Dr. Checkoway has been principal investigator include epidemiologic studies of cancer mortality in nuclear workers, cancer mortality in phosphate industry workers, silicosis and lung cancer in silica-exposed diatomaceous earth industry workers, lung cancer among chromate-exposed aerospace workers, reproductive hazards among lead smelter workers, and environmental and genetic risk factors for Parkinson's disease.

R. J. MICHAEL FRY, M.D., is retired from Oak Ridge National Laboratory, having been head of the Cancer Section of the Biology Division. He continues to serve as consultant to the Life Sciences Division of the laboratory and as adjunct professor at the University of Tennessee. He holds M.B., B.Ch., and M.D. degrees from the University of Dublin, Ireland. Previous appointments include senior scientist in the Division of Biology and Medicine, Argonne National Laboratory, and professor in the Department. of Radiology, University of Chicago. He was editor of *Radiation Research* and continues as a consulting editor. His research focused on the effects—in particular, carcinogenesis—of ionizing and ultraviolet radiation. He is a member of International Commission on Radiological Protection's Committee 1; National Council on Radiation Protection and Measurements' Committees 1, 4, 7, 75, and 88; and chairman of the National Research Council's Board on Radiation Effects Research. His awards include the Failla and Hartman medals and the Lauriston Taylor lectureship.

SAMUEL HELLMAN, M.D., is the A.N. Pritzker Distinguished Service Professor, Department of Radiation and Cellular Oncology, University of Chicago, Center for Advanced Medicine, Chicago, Illinois. Dr. Hellman previously served as Dean and A.N. Pritzker Professor of the Division of Biological Sciences and the Pritzker School of Medicine and vice president for the Medical Center; physician-in-chief of the Memorial Sloan Kettering Hospital for Cancer and Allied Diseases; the Benno C. Schmidt Chair in Clinical Oncology at Memorial Sloan-Kettering Cancer Center; and professor of radiation oncology at Cornell University Medical College. At Harvard Medical School, Dr. Hellman served as chairman of the Department of Radiation Therapy; the Alvin T. and Viola D. Fuller American Cancer Society Professor; and director of the Joint Center for Radiation Therapy. Dr. Hellman has been active in both clinical and laboratory investigation including studies of breast cancer, prostate cancer, lymphoma, and the cell kinetics of the hematopoietic system. He is the author or co-author of some 258 scientific articles; co-editor of the standard textbook on cancer, *Cancer: Principles and Practice of Oncology,* and co-editor of "The Cancer Journal" from *Scientific American.* Dr. Hellman served as chairman of the board of Allegheny College (1987-1993), where he received his B.S. degree Magna Cum Laude in 1955; is a fellow of the Institute of Medicine of the National Academy of Sciences and the American Association for the Advancement of Science; and is a member of the board of directors of Varian Associates, Inc., and of the board of trustees of The Brookings Institution. He has served as president of both the American Society for Therapeutic Radiology and Oncology and the American Society of Clinical Oncology. He received the 1980 Richard and Hinda Rosenthal Foundation Award for Clinical Research of the American Association of Cancer Research; the Gold Medals of both the American Society of Therapeutic Radiology and Oncology and the del Regato Foundation; the American Society of Therapeutic Radiology and Oncology Centennial Hartman Orator Medal; and the Claudius Regaud Medal of the European Society for Therapeautic Radiology and Oncology.

ELAINE RON, Ph.D., is chief of the Radiation Epidemiology Branch in the Division of Cancer Epidemiology and Genetics at the National Cancer Institute. Her research focuses on the carcinogenic effects of radiation exposure and the epidemiology of thyroid cancer. She is a consultant to the United Nations Scientific Committee on the Effects of Atomic Radiation (UNSCEAR) and an adviser to the National Council on Radiation Protection and Measurements' Committee 1-8 on Induction of Thyroid Cancer by Ionizing Radiation. She is a fellow of the American Epidemiology Society and a member of the Society for Epidemiologic Research and the Radiation Research Society. Dr. Ron holds a master's degree in health service administration from Yale University and a Ph.D. in epidemiology from Tel Aviv University. She currently is an associate editor of *Radiation Research.*

WILLIAM G. SEIBERT, M.A., is the senior archivist at the National Archives and Records Administration's Military Personnel Records facility in St. Louis. He has worked with NARA's collections of twentieth century military personnel and medical records for 20 years and has wide knowledge of alternate record sources available for use in reconstructing military service and medical data on individuals whose records were lost in the 1973 St. Louis fire. Mr. Seibert is a member of the Academy of Certified Archivists. He holds a B.A. in history from the College of William and Mary and a B.A. and M.A. in law from the University of Oxford.

JOHN E. TILL, Ph.D. Following graduation with distinction from the U.S. Naval Academy in 1967, Dr. John Till served in the U.S. Navy Nuclear Submarine Program. He has received the E.O. Lawrence Award from the U.S. Department of Energy in the field of environmental science and technology for his work in public involvement and research in dose reconstruction and the Elda E. Anderson Award from the Health Physics Society. He received his Ph.D. degree from the Georgia Institute of Technology in 1976, worked as a staff scientist at the Oak Ridge National Laboratory, and in 1977 formed Radiological Assessments Corporation. Renamed the Risk Assessment Corporation in 1998, it conducts independent research concerning environmental risk analysis for radionuclides and chemicals, playing a key role in the evolution of methodologies for environmental risk analysis. Dr. Till's scientific achievements include more than 150 publications, including editing the first textbook on radiation dose analysis, *Radiological Assessment*, and other documents that stress new approaches to apply and simplify risk analysis. Dr. Till's current work focuses on the assessment of risk from past releases of radionuclides and chemicals. He has been responsible for the dosimetry estimates in a major University of Utah epidemiologic dose reconstruction project, supported by the National Cancer

Institute, and was chairman of the Technical Steering Panel that directed the Hanford Environmental Dose Reconstruction Project. In this capacity, he led an effort to actively involve the public in scientific research to determine the effects of early Hanford environmental contaminants. He is a member of Committee 4 of the International Commission on Radiological Protection and the National Council on Radiation Protection and Measurements. He also serves on numerous national and international committees and advisory groups.

CLARICE R. WEINBERG, Ph.D., is currently chief of the Biostatistics Branch at the National Institute of Environmental Health Sciences, National Institutes of Health. She is also adjunct professor in the Department of Epidemiology and the Department of Biostatistics at the University of North Carolina, Chapel Hill. She holds a master's in mathematics from Brandeis University and a Ph.D. in biostatistics from the University of Washington. Her areas of expertise are reproductive epidemiology, modeling of human fertility, and statistical methods in epidemiology. She is a fellow of the American Statistical Association, an editor at the *American Journal of Epidemiology*, and serves on the editorial boards of *Epidemiology and Environmental Health Perspectives.*